MILADY STANDARD COSMETOLOGY

Haircutting

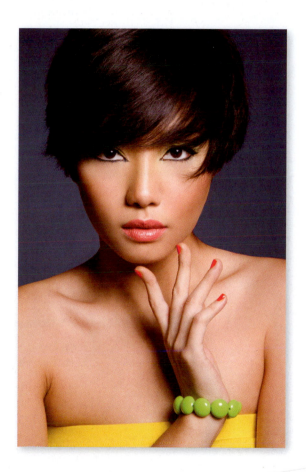

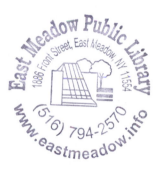

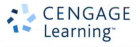
CENGAGE
Learning™

Australia • Brazil • Japan • Korea • Mexico • Singapore • Spain • United Kingdom • United States

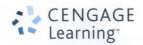

Milady Standard Cosmetology: Haircutting
Frank Shipman, Maura Scali-Sheahan

President, Milady: Dawn Gerrain

Director of Content & Business Development:
Sandra Bruce

Associate Acquisitions Editor: Philip Mandl

Product Manager: Maria Moffre-Barnes

Editorial Assistant: Elizabeth A. Edwards

Director of Marketing & Training:
Gerard McAvey

Marketing Manager: Matthew McGuire

Senior Production Director: Wendy A. Troeger

Production Manager: Sherondra Thedford

Senior Content Project Manager:
Angela Sheehan

Technology Director: Sandy Charette

Senior Art Director: Benjamin Gleeksman

For product information and technology assistance, contact us at
Professional & Career Group Customer Support, 1-800-648-7450

For permission to use material from this text or product,
submit all requests online at **cengage.com/permissions**.
Further permissions questions can be e-mailed to
permissionrequest@cengage.com.

Library of Congress Control Number: 2010903896

ISBN-13: 978-1-4390-5896-1

ISBN-10: 1-4390-5896-2

Milady
Executive Woods
5 Maxwell Drive
Clifton Park, NY 12065
USA

Cengage Learning is a leading provider of customized learning solutions with office locations around the globe, including Singapore, the United Kingdom, Australia, Mexico, Brazil, and Japan. Locate your local office at **www.cengage.com/global**

Cengage Learning products are represented in Canada by Nelson Education, Ltd.

To learn more about Milady, visit **milady.cengage.com**

Purchase any of our products at your local college store or at our preferred online store **www.cengagebrain.com**

Printed in China
3 4 5 6 7 16 15 14 13

Table of Contents

Preface

Milady Standard Cosmetology: Haircutting is a full-color, spiral-bound supplement to the leading cosmetology textbook, *Milady Standard Cosmetology*. This workbook provides you with step-by-step technical procedures for Women's Haircutting and Hairstyling and for Men's Haircutting. Each technical element features two components: an overview and procedure. The overview is a short introduction providing a framework about the technique you will learn. The procedure is the step-by-step section of the technique. Each step is explained in detail and is accompanied throughout by photos. All procedures end with photos of the same technique performed on different hair lengths, colors, and textures to help ignite your imagination. This will help you consider different possibilities for applying what you've learned in many creative ways.

WOMEN'S HAIRCUTTING

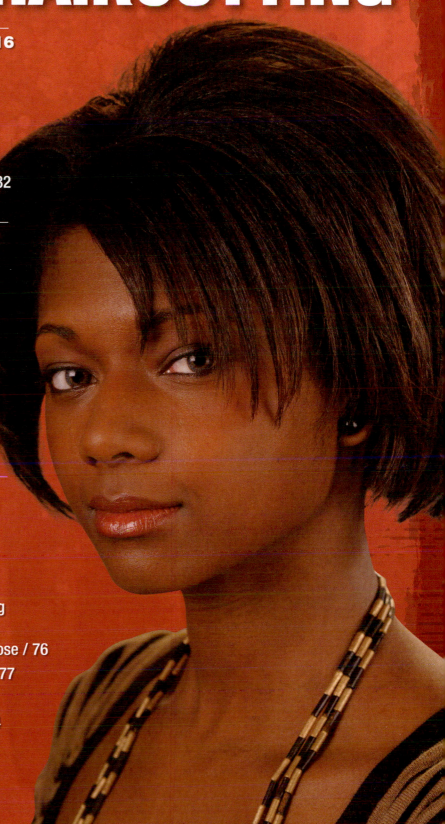

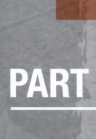

PART

The Blunt Haircut

The blunt cut has many names: *Solid Form, One Length, Zero Elevation,* and *Bob*, to name a few. The blunt cut is recognized as an all-time classic. Prior to the twentieth century, all training and emphasis was on the arrangement and curling of long hair. With World War I came change—women left the home and entered the work place, full dresses and the inconvenience of long hair no longer fit. In 1915 Irene Castle, a famous dancer of the time, introduced her *Castle Bob*; the hairstyle was adopted by film stars Colleen Moore and Louise Brooks shortly after in the early 1920s. It was seen as shocking to many, but quickly became popular among independent young women. The clean lines and easy care of the *bob* typified the modern age and the Industrial Revolution. With the 1930s came a longer length and the introduction of Marcel waves and curls. By the 1940s, layers and more extensive styling were on the rise. Not until the 1960s with the rise of the Women's Liberation Movement, the Beatles, and Vidal Sassoon, did the bob or blunt cut become popular again. It has become recognized as a classic cut of sophistication and class.

An important note is that for all the updates, trends, and variations, the original lines always look current and in style. The blunt haircut is adaptable to most textures, face shapes, and body types. With straight hair it contours to the curve of the head, neck, and shoulders; has minimal volume; and yet offers movement. Add texture or curl and the silhouette takes on a completely different look—it has increased volume and an expanded shape; the surface consists of waves with curly ends.

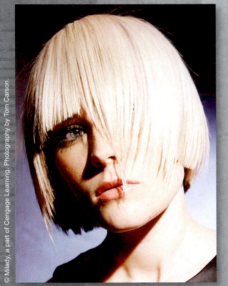

An extreme example is 1970s comedian Gilda Radner's *Saturday Night Live* character, Rosanne Roseannadanna. Although the line of the cut appears to be simple, the success of the cut relies on precision, which can be anything but simple when working with a variety of hair types, growth patterns, and animated clients.

Here we will explore a couple of variations of the classic Bob.

© Milady, a part of Cengage Learning. Photography by Tom Carson.

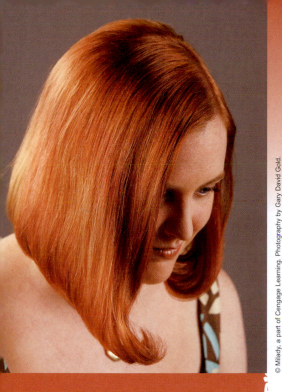

Diagonal Forward Blunt Haircut

Implements and Materials

You will need all of the following implements, materials, and supplies:

- **Cutting cape**
- **Cutting or styling comb**
- **Haircutting shears**
- **Neck strip**
- **Sectioning clips**
- **Spray bottle with water**
- **Towels**
- **Wide-tooth comb**

Overview

A true classic, this cut was first introduced by Vidal Sassoon and was later referred to as the *A-line* or *Bias-line*. The dynamic diagonal line gives this cut a swingy, free-moving quality. The hair is cut shorter at the center back area, then lengthens as it travels to the front. The shorter hair pushes and directs the longer hair, making the A-line cut move forward. The side parting makes for an evocative and dramatic sweep of hair as it frames the face.

These technical steps follow the client consultation and shampoo service.

In the diagonal forward blunt cut, lengths progress from shortest at the crown to longest at the front hairline. All lengths fall to one level along the forward diagonal perimeter frame.

Technical Drawing

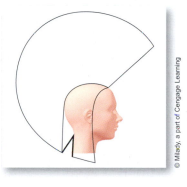

Diagonal Forward Blunt Haircut continued

Procedure

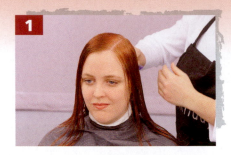

1 Establish your part and gently comb the hair into place with the client's head held upright. This cut will use a side parting. Comb all the hair into its natural falling position. Make certain the ends are combed neatly in place.

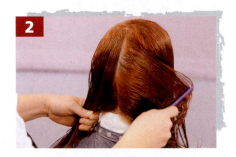

2 Part the back from the crown straight down to the nape, dividing it into two equal sections. Comb and clip the remaining hair out of the way.

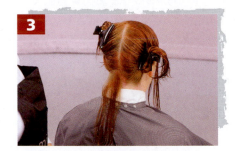

3 Take a ½-inch (1.25 cm) diagonal parting on the left side, from the center to the ear and comb it down.

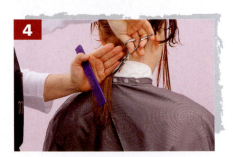

4 Begin cutting on the left side. Comb the section down with 0-degree elevation. Holding the hair straight down with the back of your left hand, angle your fingers from the center of the back to the ear, to create a diagonal, forward line. Maintain moderate tension as you cut against the neck, along the bottom of your little finger. Notice that the scissors are held palm down.

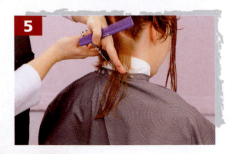

5 Move to the right side and take an identical ½-inch (1.25 cm) parting. Comb the hair down and place your hand so that it forms a diagonal, forward line. Standing just to the left of this section to allow for comfort, hold the hair with your left hand and cut with your right. Using consistent tension, cut against the neck from the center to the side. Notice that the scissors are held palm up.

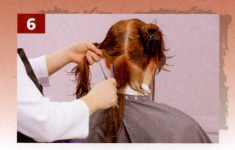

6 Return to the left side. Take down another ½-inch (1.25 cm) diagonal section and cut to match the length and angle of the previously cut section.

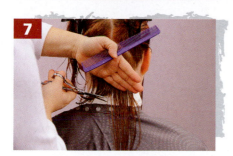

7 Repeat the procedure on the right side, again cutting the new ½-inch (1.25 cm) section to your established guideline. When you move from the left to the right side, switch from holding your scissors palm down to palm up.

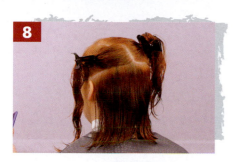

8 Continue in this manner until you reach the crest (also called the parietal ridge; it is the widest area of the head, starting at the temples and ending at the bottom of the crown). Standing in front of your client, take a diagonal parting that moves all the way from the center back, through the side, to the front. With the head straight up, comb the sides and back in their natural falling position and continue diagonal cutting from the center back toward the front.

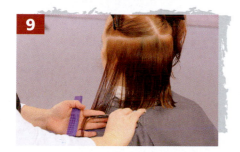

9 When you reach the ear, move toward the side. Holding the hair between your index and middle fingers, complete the diagonal forward line by bringing down subsequent ½-inch (1.25 cm) sections until the entire side is cut.

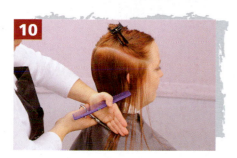

10 Move to the opposite side and repeat the procedure, bringing down ½-inch (1.25 cm) sections and cutting to establish the diagonal forward side lengths. Move the head forward as you cut the back area against the skin. Position the head upright as you cut the side area between the fingers along the diagonal forward line.

Part 1: The Blunt Haircut

Diagonal Forward Blunt Haircut continued

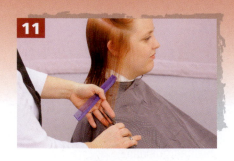

11 Continue bringing down sections until you complete the left side.

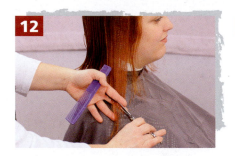

12 Complete the right side in the same manner.

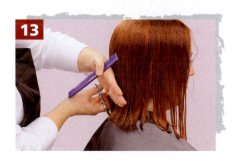

13 Check the perimeter of the cut for balance. Refine the line, if necessary.

14 The finished cut exhibits a gentle diagonal perimeter line around the face. The weight line provides for great freedom of movement.

Part 1: The Blunt Haircut

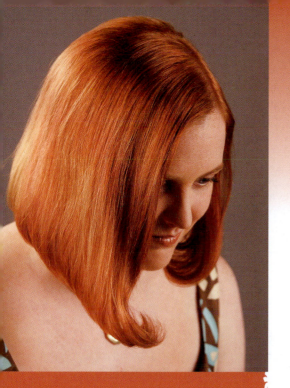

Diagonal Forward Blunt Haircut Finishing Option

© Milady, a part of Cengage Learning. Photography by Gary David Gold.

Implements and Materials

You will need all of the following implements, materials, and supplies:

- **Shampoo cape**
- **Neck strip**
- **Sectioning clips**
- **Spray bottle with water**
- **Towels**
- **Wide-tooth comb**
- **Heat-resistant rubber-based round or half-round brush**
- **Blowdryer**
- **Blowdryer nozzle**
- **Blowdryer diffuser**
- **Appropriate styling products**

Overview

This style begins with the diagonal forward blunt cut. When you style, you will maintain the neat lines of the classic blunt cut while directing more hair forward, toward the face. It is a classic look with a contemporary twist that will work for a variety of client face shapes, ages, and lifestyles.

These technical steps follow the client consultation and shampoo service.

Procedure

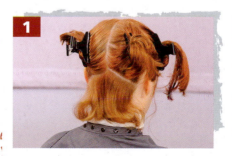

1 Part the hair from the top of the ear, over the top of the head, to the other ear and move the hair out of the way. Subdivide the back section, first down the center back, then the nape area. Part off diagonal sections on both sides, and comb and clip the upper lengths out of the way.

Diagonal Forward Blunt Haircut
Finishing Option continued

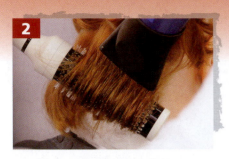

2 Starting at the nape and using a small to medium round brush, roll the hair over the brush and raise and lower the brush while following it with a blowdryer to create volume.

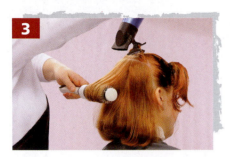

3 Continue this procedure up the back area in 1- to 1½-inch (2.5 to 3.75 cm) sections. Revolve the round brush along the lengths of the hair to create the end fullness. Use tension for the ultimate smoothing effect. Complete the entire back section in this manner.

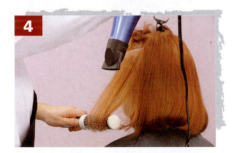

4 Move to the left side section and begin drying the hair starting with the section over the ear, then moving up toward the side part.

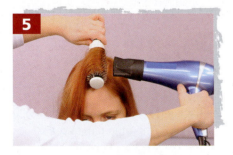

5 At the side part area, hold the section in the brush, straight out, while you blowdry the base area and continue through to the ends.

6 Switch to a smaller round or half-round brush and redefine the ends by first adding heat, then pressing the cooling button. Move to the right side and blowdry the hair in the same manner. At the side part area, hold the section and the brush straight out while you dry the base area and continue through to the ends.

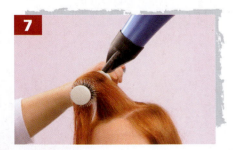

7 To create more height in the top area, hold the hair straight out from the base with a brush. First dry the base, and then continue outward through the hair lengths for added strength.

© Milady, a part of Cengage Learning. Photography by Gary David Gold.

8 Again, use a small brush to accentuate the ends. Brush and loosen the entire design.

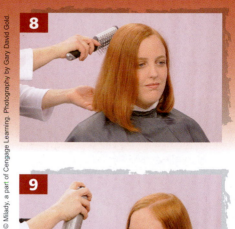

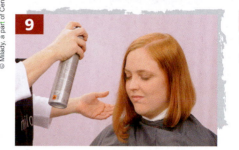

9 To finish the design, spray the top surface of the hair and smooth with your hand. The diagonal forward blunt cut with swingy voluminous movement—a modern classic!

Create

Apply this technique to different hair lengths, colors, and textures for almost endless possibilities.

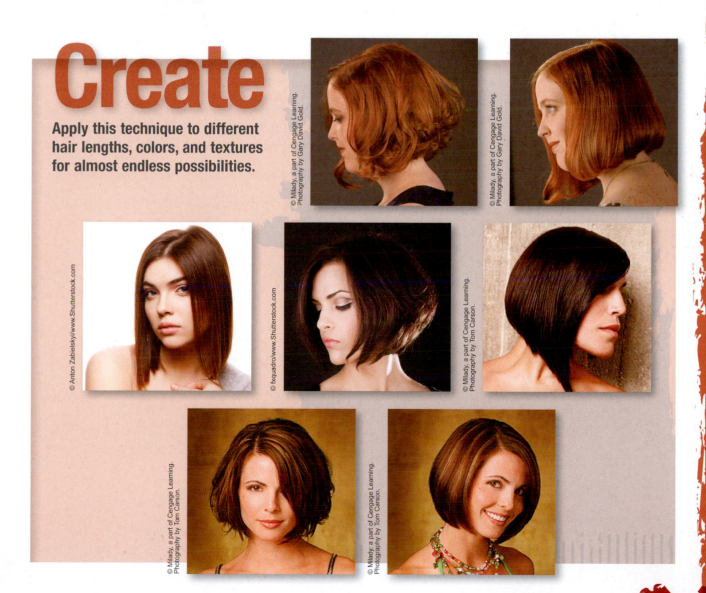

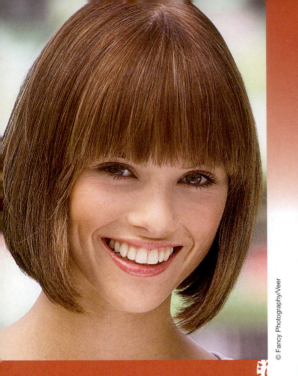
© Fancy Photography/Veer

Diagonal Back Blunt Haircut

Overview

The diagonal back blunt cut has a curvy, continuous perimeter line, creating a fluid look. Shorter at the front, then lengthening at the center back, this style—also called a *Pageboy*—provides much versatility in its styling options. The line allows for great freedom of movement, perhaps one reason why Vidal Sassoon chose this cut (originally created for the famous dancer Isadora Duncan) to reinterpret. This shorter version of the "Isadora" cut is indeed poetry in motion.

These technical steps follow the client consultation and shampoo service.

The diagonal back frame moves from just below the jaw to the collar area at the back of the head.

Technical Drawing

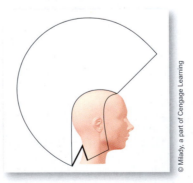
© Milady, a part of Cengage Learning

Procedure

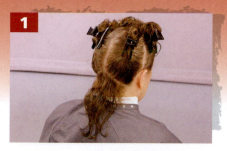

1 Begin by establishing a center part. Gently comb the hair into place with the head upright. Part the hair across the head from ear to ear. Clip side sections out of the way. Create a part down the center of the back and clip hair out of the way on both sides. Take a ½-inch (1.25 cm) parting at the nape on both sides.

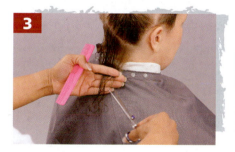

2 Position the back of your hand against the head so your fingers point down toward the nape and your wrist is slightly elevated. Using a palm-down cutting position, cut diagonally from the center back to the side.

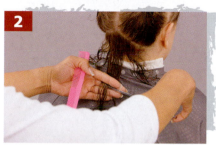

3 For the side, use the palm-up cutting position. Angle your hand by dropping your wrist, with fingers pointing toward the ear. Cut from the center back toward the side.

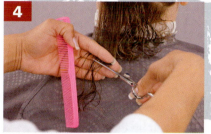

4 Return to the left side, part off another ½-inch (1.25 cm) diagonal section of hair and cut to your already established guide.

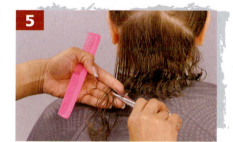

5 Continue moving side to side and cutting ½-inch (1.25 cm) diagonal sections up to the crest. Maintain 0-degree elevation, even tension, and the diagonal back cutting line.

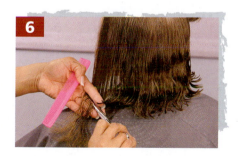

6 When you reach the crest, take a ½-inch (1.25 cm) diagonal parting that moves all the way from the center back, through the side, to the front. With the head straight up, comb the sides and back into a natural fall. Cut the side section, using your hand to continue the diagonal back line, from the back section you just cut to the front.

Diagonal Back Blunt Haircut continued

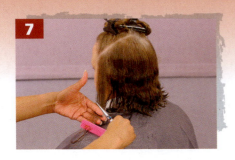

7 As you reach the front, move your body into position at the left side. Bring down subsequent sections and complete the left side.

8 Move to the right side. Take a parting from the back through the side, then cut. Use 0-degree elevation and position your hand to continue the diagonal back line.

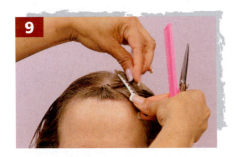

9 When you reach the recession area at the corner of the eye, clip the fringe area out of the way and complete cutting the right side.

10 Check the cut for balance, making certain both sides are cut to the same length at the same angle.

11 Release the top front area and comb it down. If side parted, push the heavy side back at the eyebrow to match the position of the hair on the opposite side. Hold the front section and cut.

12 In the finished cut, the strong diagonal back line is evident.

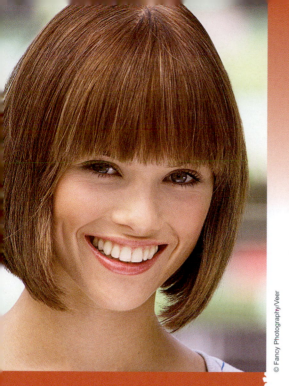

Diagonal Back Blunt Haircut Finishing Option

© Fancy Photography/Veer

Implements and Materials

You will need all of the following implements, materials, and supplies:

- **Shampoo cape**
- **Neck strip**
- **Sectioning clips**
- **Spray bottle with water**
- **Towels**
- **Wide-tooth comb**
- **Heat-resistant rubber-based round or half-round brush**
- **Blowdryer**
- **Blowdryer nozzle**
- **Blowdryer diffuser**
- **Appropriate styling products**

Overview

One of the most requested services in the salon is blowdrying hair with texture into a straight shape. This style is relatively easy—but it takes patience, the right tools, and the right styling products. Focusing on one section at a time is the key to a straight finished design.

These technical steps follow the client consultation, shampoo service, and haircut.

Procedure

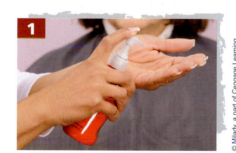

© Milady, a part of Cengage Learning. Photography by Gary David Gold.

1 Some of the styling products you can choose from are liquid gel, conditioning foam, and silicone shiner. You may even choose to combine them.

Diagonal Back Blunt Haircut
Finishing Option continued

2 Apply the product of your choice and work it through the hair.

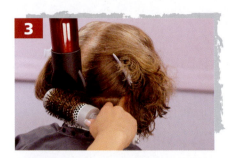

3 The hair will be divided into 1-inch (2.5 cm) sections throughout the entire head for blowdrying. Clip the upper hair neatly out of the way. Start drying at the nape area. Use a large, round bristled brush to stretch and dry the hair. This type of brush allows for extra tension.

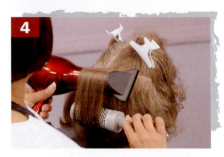

4 Use the side of the nozzle to maintain control of the section you are drying. The nozzle is inserted under the strand of hair to hold it in place when repositioning the brush.

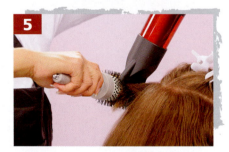

5 Follow the round brush with the blowdryer. Keep the brush and airflow moving through the hair.

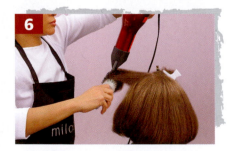

6 Use tension to stretch the top surface of the hair for a smoother finish. Move the heat over the surface of the hair more slowly than normal, because it takes more heat to straighten.

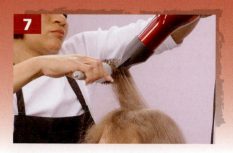

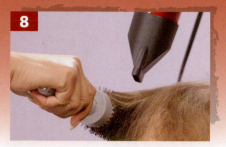

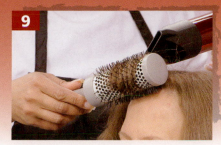

7 Holding the hair tightly, add heat to the surface of the finished style.

8 Use the cooling button on the blowdryer to help set in movement or smoothness.

9 Use the curve of the brush to add bend to the ends of the hair.

10 Smooth the hair with a wide-tooth comb. Lightly spray the shape for hold or apply a shine or gloss product to the hair's surface. The finished style has a smooth texture, which defines the diagonal back blunt shape. Curly hair has been transformed through the blowdrying technique.

Create

Apply this technique to different hair lengths, colors, and textures for almost endless possibilities.

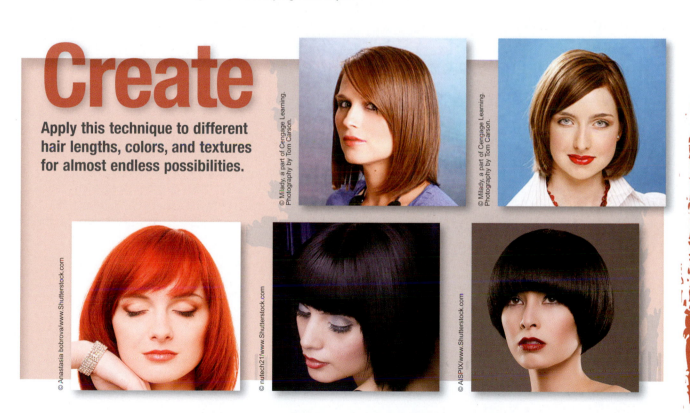

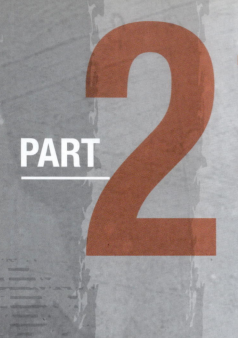

PART 2 The Graduated Haircut

The graduated cut has many names—*Bowl Cut, Wedge, Stack,* and *Emo Cut,* to name a few. The graduated cut offers a tremendous amount of movement to the wearer. The most iconic graduated cut was Dorothy Hamill's wedge cut of the 1970s. Debuting at the 1976 Winter Olympics, gold medal figure skater Dorothy Hamill's new wedge haircut fell into place perfectly with each spin on the ice and grabbed the world's attention. It became the most requested haircut in salons around the world and continues to be an important part of today's styling repertoire.

With the introduction of the graduated haircut, hairdressers were able to create inherent shape, volume, and movement. A cut could dry naturally into a style! This was the introduction of "wash and wear" hair. Also in the late 1970s came the advent of the disco era, and the graduated cut—combined with new permanent wave technology and techniques—gave hairdressers unlimited design opportunities to meet the needs of this new generation. Retro hairstyles were possible without the original style's required shampoo and set. The graduated cut has become a timeless classic with the opportunity for a trendy update through the use of a little variation. It is an invaluable cutting technique for the client with fine or thinning hair, giving them the desired look of fullness or thicker hair. Once you have a thorough understanding of graduation, the technique can be applied in combination with other cutting techniques for the creation of endless design possibilities.

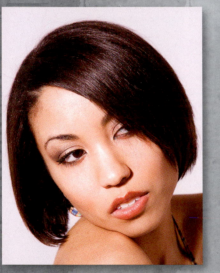

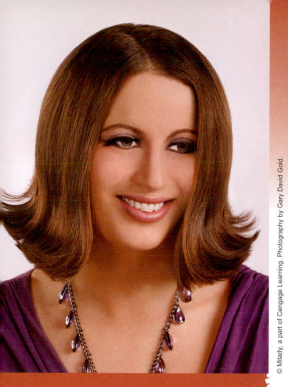

Subtle Graduated Blunt Haircut

Implements and Materials

You will need all of the following implements, materials, and supplies:

- **Cutting cape**
- **Cutting or styling comb**
- **Haircutting shears**
- **Neck strip**
- **Sectioning clips**
- **Spray bottle with water**
- **Towels**
- **Wide-tooth comb**

Overview

In this cut you will combine two distinctively different shapes in a harmonious fashion. The graduated nape area flows into a blunt diagonal forward shape toward the front and sides of the design. To create the cut, you will learn two new techniques: the use of graduation through the nape area and the use of point cutting to refine and soften the graduation as well as the perimeter line. This graduated blunt cut—some call it the graduated bob—is modern in its silhouette, and its diagonal forward line gives great freedom of movement. The close-fitting nape area is very sculptural in nature, while the rest of the cut features great structure and shape.

The graduated blunt cut is a modern classic. The sculpted graduation at the nape falls into a beautifully defined weight area at the sides.

These technical steps follow the client consultation and shampoo service.

Technical Drawing

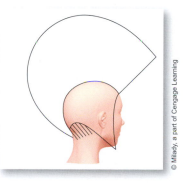

Subtle Graduated Blunt Haircut continued

Procedure

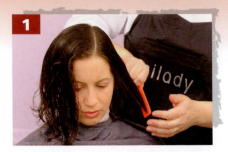

1 In this cut you will use the palm-to-palm scissor position. Prepare the hair by creating a left side part and comb the hair in its natural falling position.

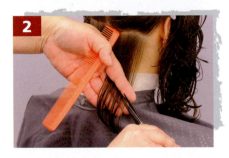

2 Move to the back of the head and take a vertical parting down the center of the back section from the top of the crown to the nape, dividing the back into two sections. On the left side, part off a 1-inch (2.5 cm) section at the nape and clip the remaining hair up and out of the way.

3 Repeat on the right side.

4 Now you will cut your guide.

5 Beginning at the back on the left side cut, comb, and elevate the hair holding it one finger's distance from the base area. This is a 30- to 45-degree elevation, or the holding position, for creating graduation.

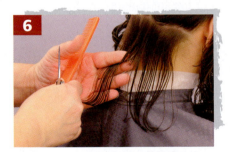

6 Cut the section diagonally along the inside of the middle finger of your left hand which is holding the hair. Notice how the entire left hand is angled downward to the left.

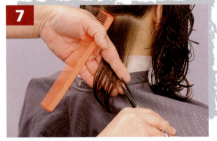

7 Repeat the procedure on the right side, cutting the hair in the opposite direction.

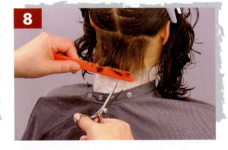

8 To refine the perimeter shape at the nape, hold the section out with your comb and use a point cutting technique.

9 When complete, the first section already shows graduation: rather than lying flat, the hair stacks along the graduated angle you have cut.

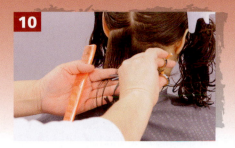

10 Release the next ½-inch (1.25 cm) section. You should be able to see the previously cut guideline through it.

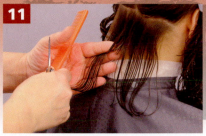

11 Comb the hair down and out at a 30-degree elevation and cut following the established guideline.

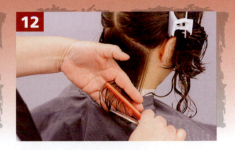

12 Repeat this procedure on the opposite side.

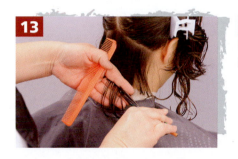

13 Continue to bring down ½-inch (1.25 cm) sections and cut to your guide. This will be the procedure as you work up the back area. Do not shift the hair away from the natural fall direction.

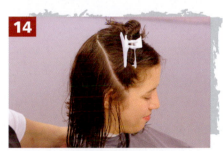

14 When you reach the crest, you will begin to work on the sides. Part all the way through the sides, taking a diagonal forward section that is no more than ½ inch (1.25 cm) over the ear. Bring the head upright. Cut diagonally with 0-degree elevation. Position your fingers to establish the length and create the diagonal line; cut the entire side section, holding the hair as close to the skin as possible.

15 Comb the hair against the skin and check the line for accuracy. This will accentuate a blunt line.

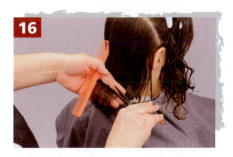

16 Move to the right side. Bring down a ½-inch (1.25 cm) diagonal parting over the ear. Bring the head upright. Holding the hair low, begin cutting at the graduated back. Cut diagonally forward with the hair in natural fall. Position your fingers to establish the length and create the diagonal line; cut the entire side section, working as close to the skin as possible.

17 Before cutting subsequent partings at the sides, check the length on both sides to make certain they are even.

Subtle Graduated Blunt Haircut continued

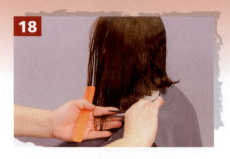

18 Return to the left side. Part out diagonally, releasing ½-inch (1.25 cm) sections. Cut, following the established guideline. Maintain the natural fall direction when working toward the sides, holding the hair at 0-degree elevation. Continue to use this technique to the top side parting.

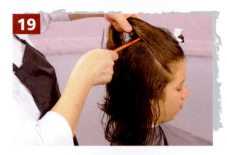

19 Continue on the right side, parting out diagonally to release sections.

20 Maintain natural fall while cutting through the sides, following the established guide. Continue to follow the established guideline to cut diagonally toward the front and sides.

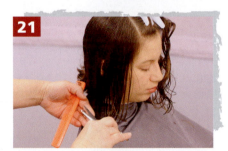

21 Move to the side and cut in natural fall.

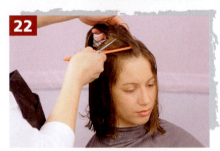

22 Section out the top front fringe area, part and comb it to the right side, and cut it at an angle through the front that blends with the sides. Cutting of the top is performed on the heavy side of the part— the right side—only.

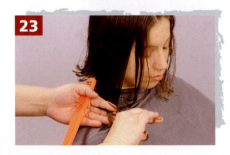

23 Check the entire perimeter using the point cutting technique. The sculptural silhouette seen here is a magnificent shape that can be adapted in a variety of ways. The precision of the shape gives the style a modern appeal.

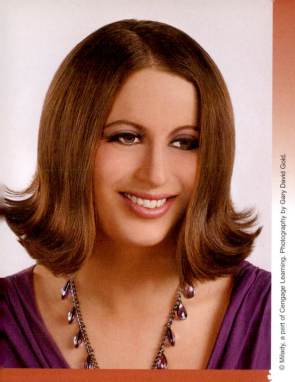

Subtle Graduated Blunt Haircut Finishing Option

Implements and Materials

You will need all of the following implements, materials, and supplies:

- **Shampoo cape**
- **Neck strip**
- **Sectioning clips**
- **Spray bottle with water**
- **Towels**
- **Wide-tooth comb**
- **Heat-resistant rubber-based vent brush**
- **Blowdryer**
- **Blowdryer nozzle**
- **Blowdryer diffuser**
- **Appropriate styling products**

Overview

This style begins after the graduated blunt cut that you completed in the haircutting procedure. Styling this cut with an asymmetric look is slimming to the face and answers the needs of the client who wants to wear a side part. The simple movement of the brush and blowdryer through the hair creates body and ornamental effects without diminishing the sculptural silhouette of the cut.

These technical steps follow the client consultation, shampoo service, and haircut.

Subtle Graduated Blunt Haircut
Finishing Option continued

Procedure

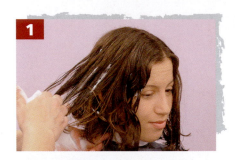

1   Apply a styling product of your choice and work it through the hair. Comb the hair into the desired shape using a side parting.

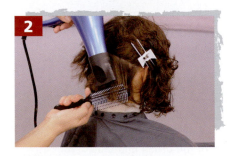

2   Begin blowdrying in the nape area with the rubber-based bristle brush. Directionally flow the hair outward from the center back on either side. The airflow follows the brush as it closely contours the hair against the head.

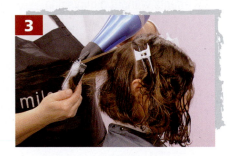

3   Above the occipital area, begin parting out along a diagonal forward. Continue upward and maintain the brush while blowdrying along the diagonal forward.

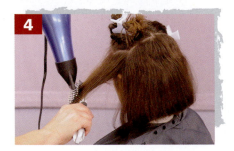

4   Continue this process into the sides and up to the side part. Lift the hair out from the base area according to the amount of base lift desired. Turn the ends and dry to bevel the ends under.

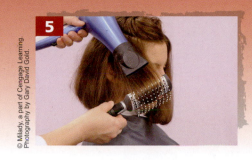

5 Finish blowdrying the front area, paying particular attention to the base area and mid-shaft. To create a smooth effect, grasp the ends in the brush and turn the ends downward.

Create

Apply this technique to different hair lengths, colors, and textures for almost endless possibilities.

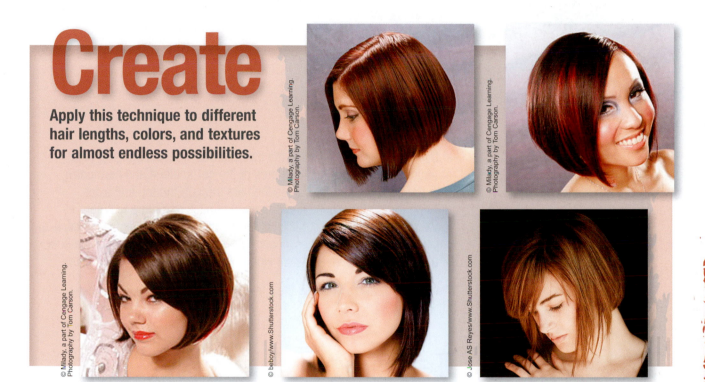

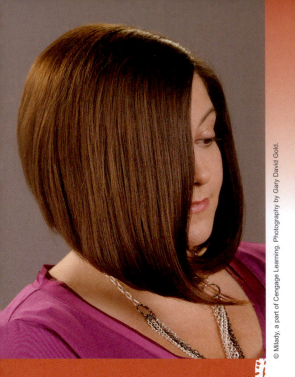

Extreme Graduated Blunt Haircut

Implements and Materials

Implements and Materials

You will need all of the following implements, materials, and supplies:

- **Cutting cape**
- **Cutting or styling comb**
- **Haircutting shears**
- **Texturizing shears**
- **Neck strip**
- **Sectioning clips**
- **Spray bottle with water**
- **Towels**
- **Wide-tooth comb**

Overview

In this style, sometimes called the Inverted Bob, you will create a high graduation throughout the back area of the cut to blend and harmonize with the blunt shape that frames the face through the top and sides. Utilizing the occipital bone and a graduated back and nape to create a forward movement, this cut is ideal for the client having a flat occipital, a weak jawline, or who wishes longer hair framing the face without the bulk of a long back. This versatile cut works well on hair of most any texture.

These technical steps follow the client consultation, shampoo service, and haircut.

Technical Drawing

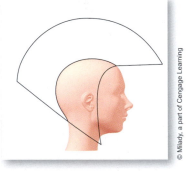

Procedure

1 In this cut we will be using the palm-to-palm shear position.

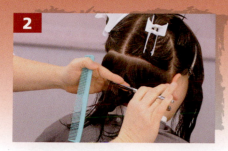

2 Prepare the hair as in blunt haircut with side part. Clip the hair in the nape section out of the way. Begin the cut in the back on the left side at the occipital bone. Take a 1-inch (2.5 cm) parting of hair at the occipital bone and comb it straight down, with a one-finger width angle. Keep in mind that the length is determined by the shape and position of the occipital bone.

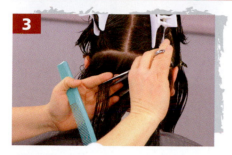
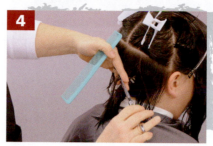
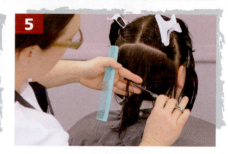

3 Cut this section diagonally along the inside of the middle finger of your left hand, which is holding the hair. The fingers of the left hand should be angled upward toward the center of the back.

4 The more angled your hand, the longer the length in the front will be. Repeat on the right side.

5 Once the left side guide has been completed, move to the right side and cut the guide in the same manner. Continue to work from side-to-side until you reach the crest area.

6 When you reach the crest, you will begin to work on the sides.

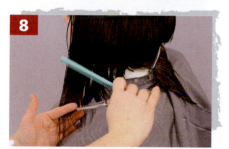

7 Take a diagonal part that extends to the front of the ear as shown. Before cutting, make sure the client's head is upright, then comb the hair into its natural fall. Position your fingers to establish the length and create the diagonal lines; cut the entire side section with little or no elevation (0 degree).

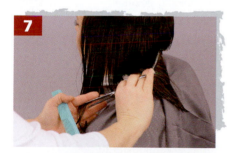

8 Comb the hair and check the line and angle for accuracy.

9 Repeat the procedure on the right side, cutting the hair in the opposite direction.

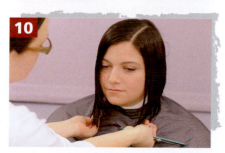

10 Before cutting below the occipital and nape area, check the length on both sides to make certain they are even.

Part 2: The Graduated Haircut

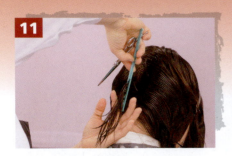

11 Move to the back and part out a ½-inch (1.25 cm) vertical section from the occipital bone to the nape.

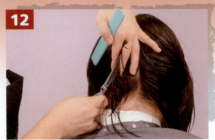

12 Starting at the top of the section, hold the hair straight out from the occipital area, angling the fingers outward from the curve of the head. Begin cutting the section, angling toward the nape.

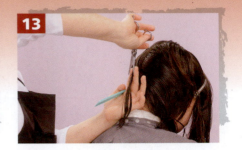

13 Continue down the section, cutting in closer to the head as you approach the nape. This will be your stationary guideline for the back.

14 Finish cutting the stationary guideline at the nape, directly below the section you just cut.

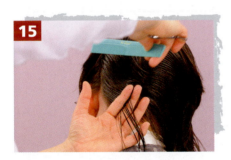

15 Part out the next vertical section and overdirect to and cut along the stationary guideline, using the same holding position and cutting angle. Continue parting and cutting vertical sections from the back to the last section behind the ear.

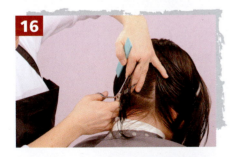

16 Move to the right side. Pick up your stationary guideline to follow. Notice the change in hand position on the right side

17 Complete each vertical section, using the same technique that you used on the left side.

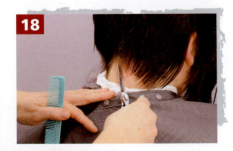

18 Refine the back and nape using a point cutting technique, cleaning up any unevenness.

19 Refine the perimeter of the cut working with the hair texture and growth patterns.

Part 2: The Graduated Haircut

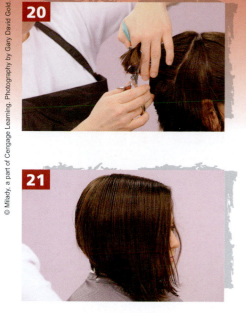

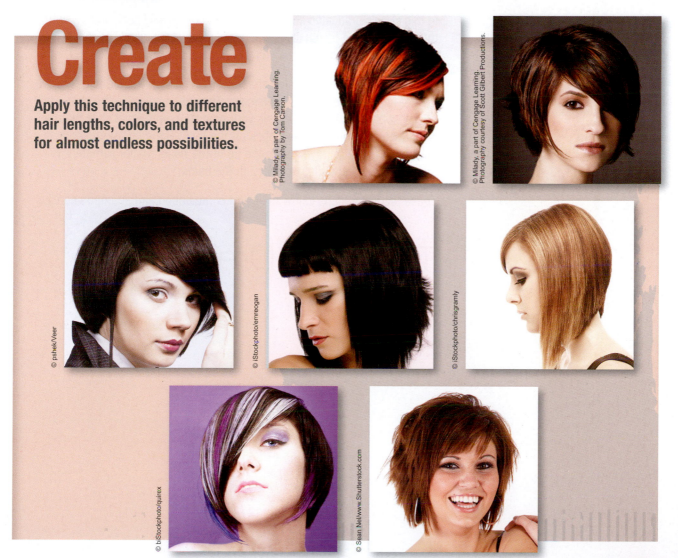

20 Soften or blend the weight line with texturizing shears.

21 The finished shape has a strong diagonal forward movement. The blunt lines of the side blend harmoniously with the graduated back area. This is a very dramatic and desirable shape to suit many clients.

Create

Apply this technique to different hair lengths, colors, and textures for almost endless possibilities.

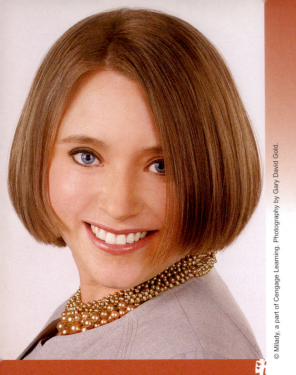

Low Graduation Haircut

Implements and Materials

You will need all of the following implements, materials, and supplies:

- **Cutting cape**
- **Cutting or styling comb**
- **Haircutting shears**
- **Neck strip**
- **Sectioning clips**
- **Spray bottle with water**
- **Towels**
- **Wide-tooth comb**

Overview

In this classic graduated shape, lengths flow diagonally back and away from the face. This mid-length style is perfect for the client who likes the look of long hair but appreciates the control and manageability of a short cut.

After you create the graduated shape, you will soften the bluntness of the weight line with texturizing techniques. This will modernize the shape and create softly rounded edges. This very popular, commercial style features a graduated frame that flows back off the face. The mid-length shape features a line that travels from the tip of the nose to approximately 1 inch (2.5 cm) below the nape area in the back.

These technical steps follow the client consultation and shampoo service.

Technical Drawing

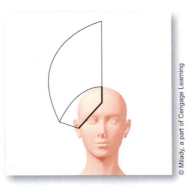

Procedure

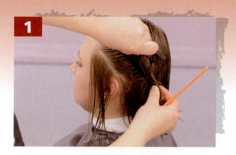

1 Establish a side part, combing the hair into natural fall with the head upright. Make sure the ends are neatly combed and comb any longer lengths back over the ear. Diagonally part a ½-inch (1.25 cm) section just in front of the ear, moving from the front hairline back over the ear.

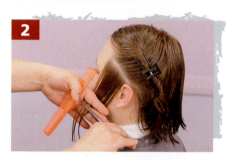

2 Use a 30-degree elevation. Angle the fingers holding the hair from the tip of the nose to the ear lobe. Use the palm-to-palm scissor position as you cut.

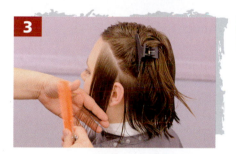

3 This diagonally angled line will be your cutting guide. Notice that it angles down from the nose to the ear lobe.

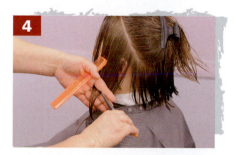

4 Part off the next section, angling down from the hairline to the back, so the part line falls ½ inch (1.25 cm) above the top of the ear. Comb the hair into the natural fall direction and cut on the diagonal, following the established guideline.

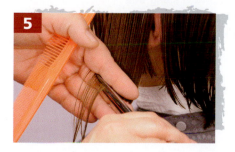

5 Hold your scissors at a low elevation in a palm-to-palm position. Taking care not to cut past your second knuckle, cut the guide, moving through to the back.

Part 2: The Graduated Haircut

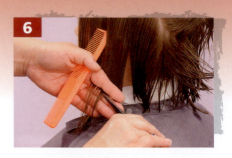

6 Continue bringing down ½-inch (1.25 cm) sections and cutting to the previous guideline. (Make certain you can see the guide through each new section.) Cut exactly on your guideline.

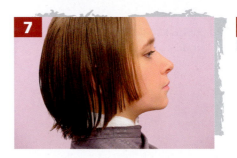

7 The completed sections should form a perfect diagonal line from front to back.

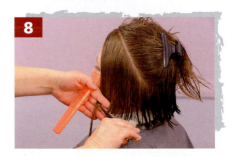

8 Complete the entire side, diagonally parting out ½-inch (1.25 cm) sections and following the guide. Maintain a 30-degree elevation. Comb the lengths against the skin and refine the perimeter line. Comb the line between the fingers and point cut to blend and refine the back area.

9 Move to the opposite side. Establish a guide as described in step 3. Cut subsequent sections as in steps 5 through 8 until you reach the recession area.

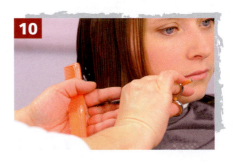

10 Part from the center front hairline to the last section cut and combine both into their natural falling position. Notice that the front hairline is left out. Cut through from the side to the nape. Blend and cut the fringe in natural fall. The horizontal finger position is aligned with the tip of the nose. Continue working upward using this procedure. Cut the sides to the guide, then cut the top front to the guide. Remember to use the natural fall direction and low elevation.

11 Comb all the top hair and front fringe down in the natural fall direction. Here you will see the guideline through the final front section.

12 Cut the fringe line to adapt to the needs and desires of your client.

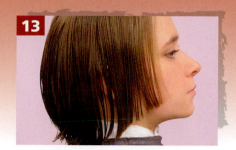

13 The completed side shows that the front piece extends toward the tip of the nose.

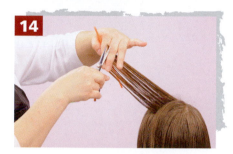

14 If you wish to soften the weight line by removing the corner, work gradually through the interior, bringing sections up and out and taking the weight corner off. You can do this by cutting blunt, pointed, or notched lines into the section.

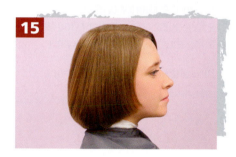

15 The graduated diagonal back silhouette flows into a softly rounded back area. The weight area, having been rounded, creates a soft shape.

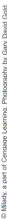

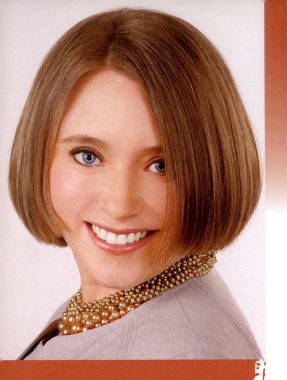

Low Graduation Haircut Finishing Option

Implements and Materials

You will need all of the following implements, materials, and supplies:

- **Shampoo cape**
- **Neck strip**
- **Sectioning clips**
- **Spray bottle with water**
- **Towels**
- **Wide-tooth comb**
- **Heat-resistant rubber-based round brush and paddle brush**
- **Blowdryer**
- **Blowdryer nozzle**
- **Blowdryer diffuser**
- **Appropriate styling products**

Overview

Styling this haircut using radial sections through the interior of the head makes the blowdrying of graduated shapes fast, easy, and efficient. You will use both the round and paddle brush to get the most volume for this style.

These technical steps follow the client consultation, shampoo service, and haircut.

Procedure

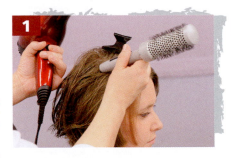

1 Apply a styling product of your choice and work it through the hair. Use a round brush to part the hair into diagonal sections through the interior.

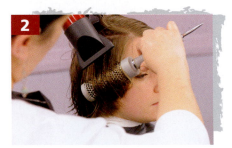

2 Work around the head using the blowdryer to follow the round brush positioned diagonally.

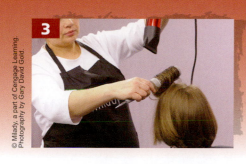

3 In the top area, direct lengths forward, rolling back toward the base while blowdrying. This will maximize volume given the overdirected base. Continue this technique toward the front hairline area. The front fringe section is rolled using the same technique to create a volume effect in this area.

4 Use a paddle brush to stretch the shape and allow airflow, brush into place.

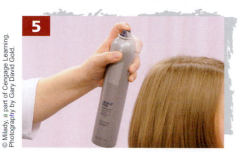

5 Use a hair spray and blowdryer technique to finish the design. Spray directionally up and into the front hairline lengths while following with the blowdryer. This will create enhanced directional hold, body, and lift. The finished style is always in fashion and wearable for a large number of clientele. The technique may be adapted on a variety of other haircuts.

Create

Apply this technique to different hair lengths, colors, and textures for almost endless possibilities.

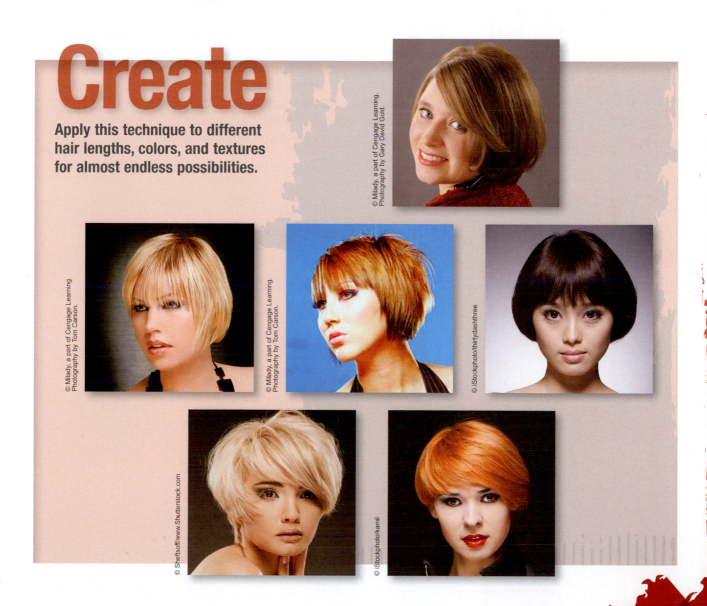

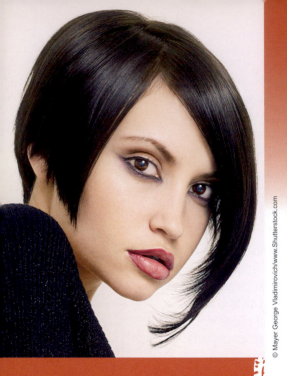

© Mayer George Vladimirovich/www.Shutterstock.com

High Graduation Haircut

Implements and Materials

You will need all of the following implements, materials, and supplies:

- Cutting cape
- Cutting or styling comb
- Haircutting shears
- Neck strip
- Sectioning clips
- Spray bottle with water
- Towels
- Wide-tooth comb

Overview

In this style, you will create high graduation throughout the entire back area of the cut to blend and harmonize with the layered shape that frames the face through the top and sides. This cut defines the head shape through the back area by the closer contours of the graduation; the layered lengths around the face frame it attractively, adding a soft, feminine touch as well as versatility. This versatile shape combines a high graduation through the back with soft layers that frame the face.

These technical steps follow the client consultation and shampoo service.

Technical Drawing

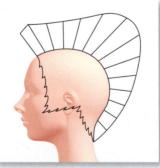

© Milady, a part of Cengage Learning

Procedure

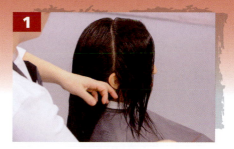

1 Create a side part and comb the hair around the curve of the head in natural fall. Part the hair across the top of the head from ear to ear and clip hair out of the way.

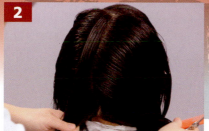

2 Move to the back and part out a ½-inch (1.25 cm) vertical section from crown to nape.

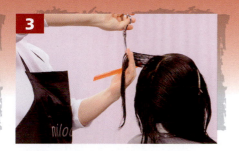

3 Starting at the top of the section, hold the hair straight back from the crown area, angling the fingers outward from the curve of the head. Begin cutting along the section, angling toward the nape.

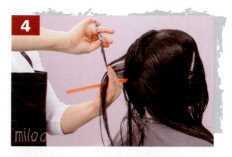

4 Continue down the section, cutting in closer to the head as you approach the nape. This will be your traveling guideline for the top and sides. Notice the holding position, straight out from the curve of the head and angled toward the nape, as you work from the crest area down.

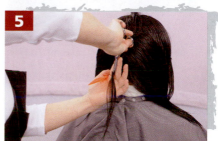

5 Finish cutting your guide to the nape, directly below the section you just cut.

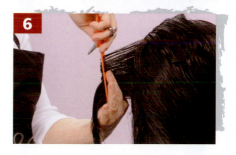

6 Moving to the left side, part out the next vertical section and take a small portion of the first section you cut (the guideline), hold it with the next vertical section and cut using the same holding position and cutting angle. Continue parting and cutting vertical sections, moving from the back toward the sides, cutting sections to the same angle as the traveling guideline. Let the guide travel slightly toward the new section being cut.

High Graduation Haircut continued

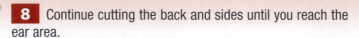

7 Take vertical subsections, in a pie shape, to take the curve of the head into account. Cut the first subsection by pulling the hair straight out from the curve of the head, cutting from the top section toward the nape.

8 Continue cutting the back and sides until you reach the ear area.

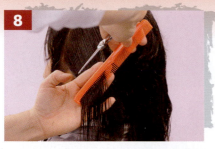

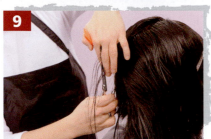

9 The last back section that you cut, which is behind the ear, will now serve as a stationery guideline to which you will bring all the side lengths. Hold the section above the ear straight out from the curve of the head. Direct all side lengths back to this guideline, section by section, and cut along the pre-established line. This will create the layered effect through the front.

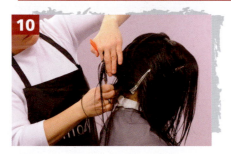

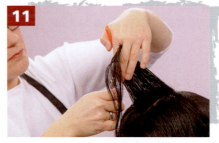

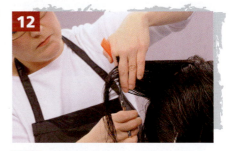

10 Move to the right side. Pick up your traveling guideline to follow. Note the change in hand and cutting position.

11 Complete each vertical section, using the same technique that you used on the first side.

12 The vertical sections that you are cutting radiate around the head. Make sure you follow your traveling guideline, which should be visible at all times.

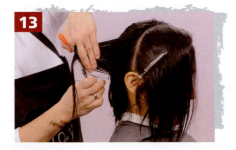

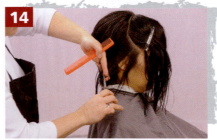

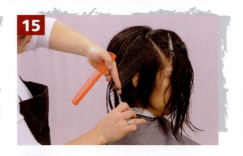

13 Stop using a traveling guideline when you reach the ear area, as you did on the first side.

14 At this point, you will switch to a stationery guideline, as you did before. Bring sections back to this guide.

15 Continue using the stationery guideline to cut the remainder of the side, bringing ½-inch (1.25 cm) sections back to it.

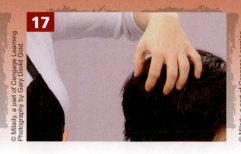

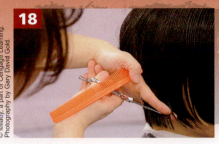

16 Bring top sections back to the crown to check and blend internal lengths across the top of the head. Cross-check throughout the cut, cleaning up any unevenness.

17 In the finished cut, graduated effects make for much textural movement.

18 Refine the perimeter of the cut, working with the facial shape and hair texture. A slicing technique is used here to soften the perimeter line.

---

19 The finished shape has a diffused softness to it. The face-framing layers blend harmoniously with the graduated back area. This is a versatile and desirable shape to suit a multitude of clients.

Create

Apply this technique to different hair lengths, colors, and textures for almost endless possibilities.

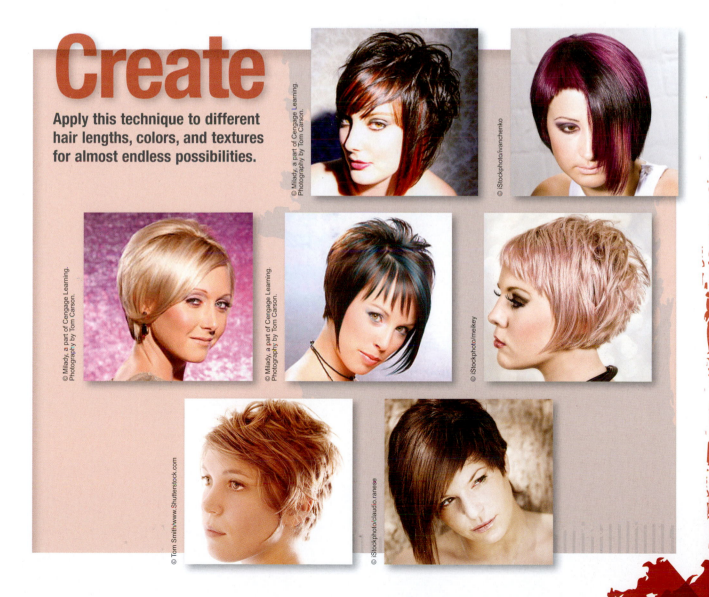

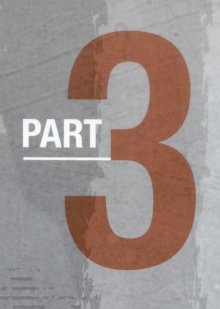

PART 3

The Layered Haircut

The layered cut is the most popular and versatile of all cuts. *The Rachel, Farrah, Mullet, Pixie, Shag,* and *Afro* are just a few of the layered cuts that defined an era and have become a classic style of today. The 1950s introduced many hairstyles that required layering. It was during the new social freedoms of the 1960s—from women's lib, civil rights, to the Summer of Love with Woodstock and the hippies—that natural hair or a more natural look became popular. The 70s "gypsy" shag was the perfect complement to the Bohemian peasant-fashion influences of the time. As always, celebrity hairstyles drove the public into salons to request the look. Audrey Hepburn, Mia Farrow, and Halle Berry (decades apart) influenced many women to cut their hair short into pixie cuts. Long-haired celebrities such as Jennifer Aniston and Farrah Fawcett had iconic long hairstyles that were desired by many young women of each star's era.

The layered cut lends volume, decreases weight, and adds internal texture and movement. These design factors are critical when considering the natural hair and desired style. What is unique to the layered cut is that it is a classic with no one particular defining look.

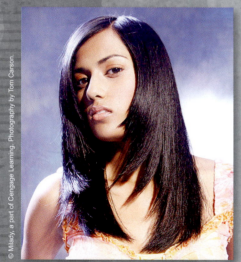

© Milady, a part of Cengage Learning. Photography by Tom Carson.

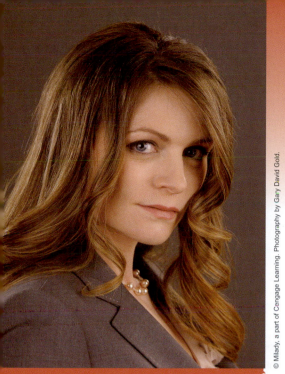

Perimeter Layers Haircut

Implements and Materials

You will need all of the following implements, materials, and supplies:

- **Cutting cape**
- **Cutting or styling comb**
- **Haircutting shears**
- **Neck strip**
- **Sectioning clips**
- **Spray bottle with water**
- **Towels**
- **Wide-tooth comb**

Overview

Long, layered shapes are an often-requested design in the salon. They are highly commercial and can be styled for a wide variety of looks. Soft, face-framing layers complement the long horizontal bluntness of the remainder of the cut.

To begin, you will learn a fundamental approach to this cut. As you progress, you will start to introduce some of the many variations on this silhouette into your work. This shape features a horizontal blunt perimeter line combined with long, soft layers that flow from the jawline down to the blunt weight line.

These technical steps follow the client consultation and shampoo service.

Technical Drawing

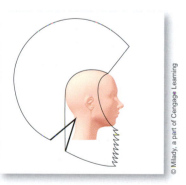

Perimeter Layers Haircut continued

Procedure

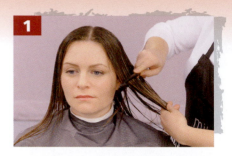

1 Establish a center part and make certain the hair is evenly distributed all around the head in natural fall.

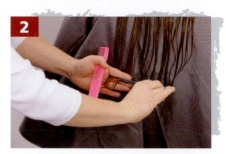

2 Begin the cut by removing excess length in the back, starting on the left back side. Use a horizontal cutting position; hold all the hair between your fingers and cut. You can also hold the hair flat with your comb and cut, using comb control alone.

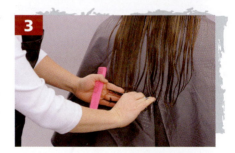

3 Cut toward the side, using the horizontal cutting position with your palm downward. Complete this side.

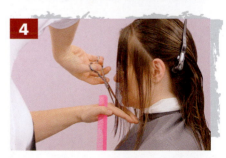

4 Continue cutting horizontally toward the front right, following the same procedure. Part off a section that moves along the hairline from the center part along with the front hairline in front of the ears and clip the remaining hair out of the way. Hold this section of the hair downward between the first and middle fingers of your hand at the jawline. Angle the fingers diagonally with the tips of the scissors, point cutting toward the chin.

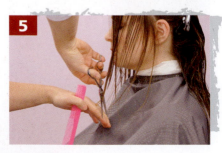

5 With your other hand, hold your scissors against the hand with the hair and begin to slide both hands down in unison as you open and close the blades along the hair to remove length. Continue moving steadily downward, making certain you maintain natural fall. Stop when you reach the bottom weight line of your perimeter. This shape is highly desirable for many clients. The possible variations with this slide-cutting technique allow for the creation of a multitude of effects.

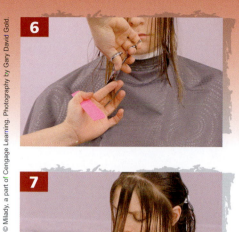

6 Cut the opposite side in the same manner, layering the hair by sliding your scissors down the entire front perimeter as you open and close the blades. Note the holding, cutting, and scissor positions being used.

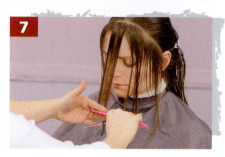

7 Cross-check the two sides for evenness, parting off a small, horizontal section at the front, combing it down, and making sure the two sides meet at the same point and blend. To create a looser, more highly textured effect, take the same partings as instructed above, but comb and elevate the hair forward. Cut the hair diagonally, slide cutting as before. More layers will result.

8 Finish as desired. The finished shape will result in soft face-framing layers that will blend into the blunt haircut.

Create

Apply this technique to different hair lengths, colors, and textures for almost endless possibilities.

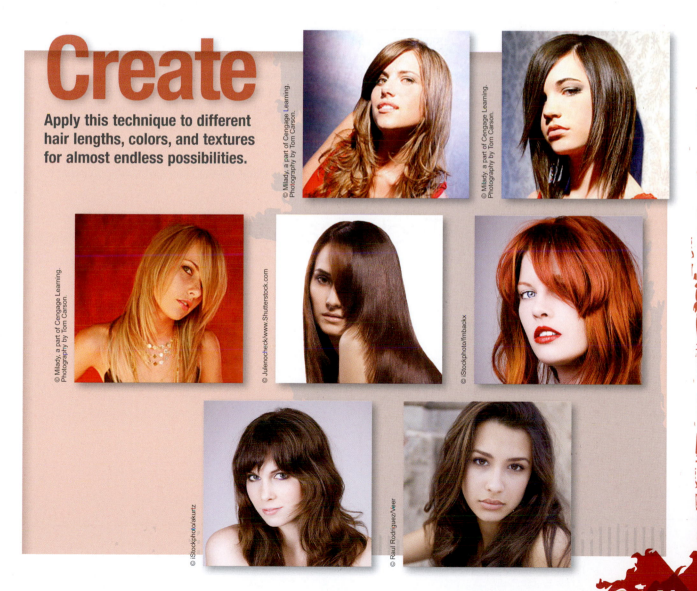

Part 3: The Layered Haircut

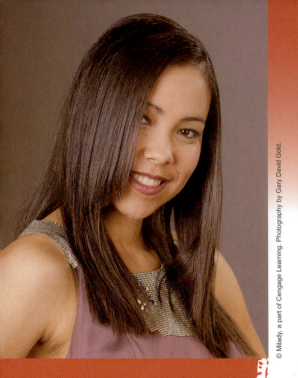

Light Layers Haircut

Implements and Materials

You will need all of the following implements, materials, and supplies:

- **Cutting cape**
- **Cutting or styling comb**
- **Haircutting shears**
- **Neck strip**
- **Sectioning clips**
- **Spray bottle with water**
- **Towels**
- **Wide-tooth comb**

Overview

This shape is a true classic—and yet very contemporary as well! Internal layers flow over the perimeter blunt cut. The longer layers in this cut are preplanned according to the initial guideline that you create around the front hairline; you will bring all internal layers to this length. The use of this stationery guide will make for shorter layers around the front hairline, increasing to longer layers at the crown and back of the head. This haircut features long or "light" layers that flow over the blunt perimeter line. More layers frame the front area, with a lesser amount of layers in the center back of the head.

These technical steps follow the client consultation and shampoo service.

Technical Drawing

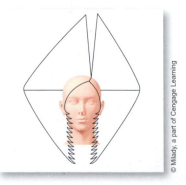

Procedure

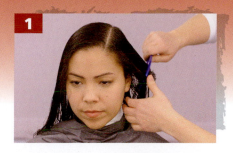

1 This haircut begins with the perimeter already cut at a zero-degree elevation. Now, establish a side part for this hairstyle. Comb the hair in natural fall.

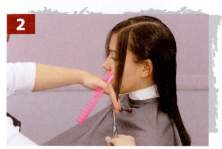

2 Locate the natural fringe area by parting a triangular section from the side part to the recession area, at the outside corner of the eye. Part off a ½-inch (1.25 cm) horizontal section from the front and clip the remainder of the section out of the way. Use a point of reference on the face, such as the lip, for where you will begin cutting on the diagonal from front to back.

3 Beginning on the left side, direct the hair in natural fall and position your fingers diagonally; position the scissors to follow the same diagonal line your fingers form. Begin cutting near the lip and follow the angle of your fingers. Cut the entire fringe section to this guide.

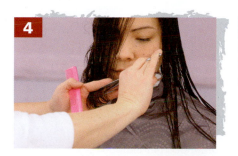

4 Repeat this procedure on the opposite side of the part. Pick up the hair at the recession area of the right side. Cut diagonally from the lip line on the diagonal from front to back, just as you did before.

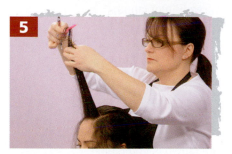

5 Part out a rectangular section through the interior of the head. Begin at the front hairline area by taking a horizontal parting from the front of the section. Hold this section straight up from the top of the head and begin cutting out diagonally about 6 inches (15 cm) from the scalp. This will be your stationery guide.

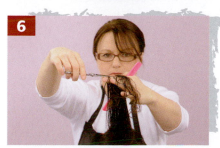

6 Hold the stationery guide straight up from the top of the head and bring partings to it as you cut on a slightly upward angle from the side part outward. Work from the front to the back of the section, taking partings and directing them to the initial stationery guide until you complete the section. This technique will create a length increase.

Part 3: The Layered Haircut

Light Layers Haircut continued

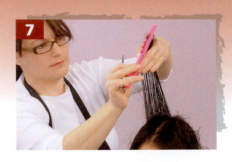

7 Cross-check these internal lengths by taking a vertical parting from the front to the crown. Note how the angle moves from shorter at the front to longer at the crown area. Direct lengths straight up and check the line.

8 Use this internal length increase as your guideline for cutting the sides. Take horizontal sections throughout the left side. Using a section of hair from the top as the guideline, bring sections straight up, distributing the hair neatly to the stationery guide, then cut to this guide along the diagonal line created.

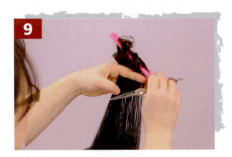

9 Moving back, bring lengths straight up to the stationery guide for cutting. Notice how the fingers of the holding hand are angled diagonally upward from front to back.

10 Continue layering one side until you run out of hair. This will be where you meet the length of the outside perimeter of the cut.

11 Move to the right side and begin bringing sections to the stationery guide and cutting diagonally. Continue cutting until this side is completed.

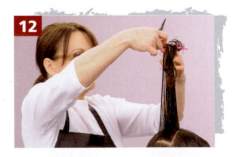

12 Blend the crown lengths into the top area. Use pie-shaped partings to work around to the back crown area. Direct lengths straight up from the top of the head and begin cutting diagonally using the predetermined length/guide from the top.

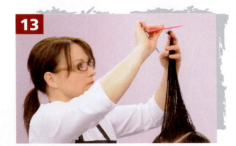

13 Continue in this manner until the entire crown is completed.

14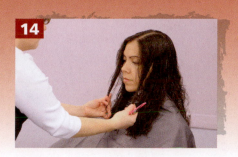

14 After completing the layering, check the hair's response by styling with your fingertips. Finish the cut by checking the line framing the face. Direct lengths forward and position the fingers outward from the fringe length cut earlier to refine the line.

15 The finished silhouette shows the long layers that have been created. These layers will allow for movement, surface texture, and dimension to be achieved in the finished style. The cut is versatile and can be styled in a variety of ways, whether back away from the face or forward onto the face.

Create

Apply this technique to different hair lengths, colors, and textures for almost endless possibilities.

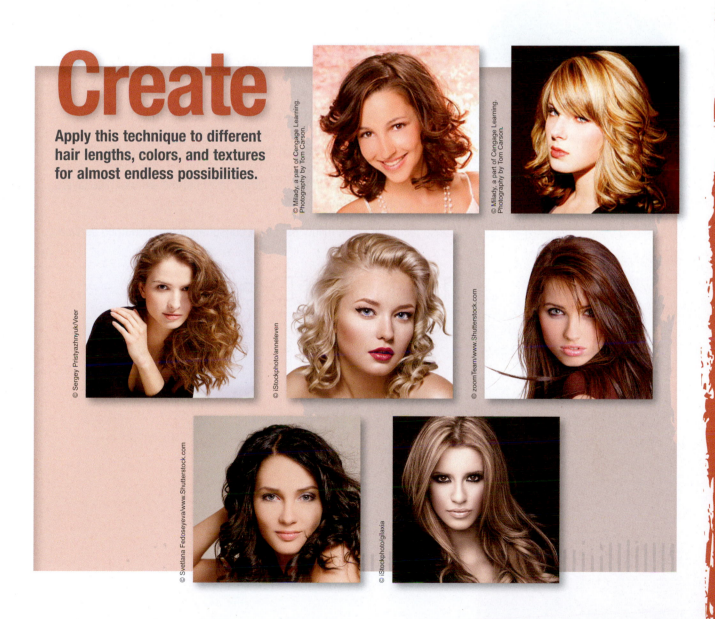

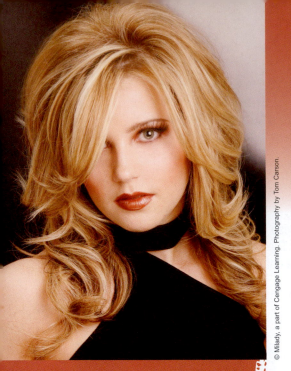

Heavy Layers Haircut on Long Hair

Implements and Materials

You will need all of the following implements, materials, and supplies:

- **Cutting cape**
- **Cutting or styling comb**
- **Haircutting shears**
- **Neck strip**
- **Sectioning clips**
- **Spray bottle with water**
- **Towels**
- **Wide-tooth comb**

Overview

This shape's heavily layered or textured effect comes from the cutting technique used throughout the interior. It can be worn straight or in a full, voluminous look; it can be styled forward or back. It provides the client with great versatility. In this heavily layered shape, lengths progress from short layers through the interior to longer layers at the exterior. The layers provide textured volume.

These technical steps follow the client consultation and shampoo service.

Technical Drawing

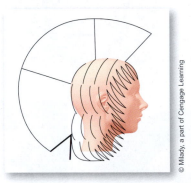

Procedure

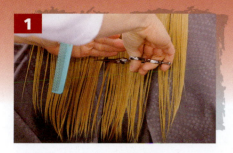

1 Begin by first establishing the perimeter length and shape. Make a center part and then take a ½-inch (1.25 cm) section along the top front hairline.

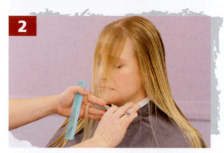

2 Comb and hold the hair downward over the face at low elevation. Use a point of reference on the face, such as the nose or chin, to establish the length, cutting horizontally.

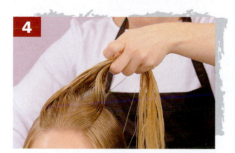

3 Section and cut the entire side hairline area. Direct and hold the hair with your fingers positioned diagonally. Cut the side lengths to blend from the fringe to the exterior length. Overdirect the hair as necessary. Repeat on the other side, cutting diagonally.

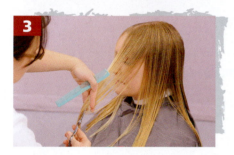

4 Part out a rectangular horizontal section through the top from the front hairline to the crown.

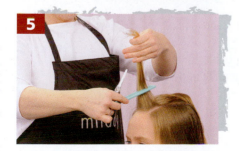

5 Hold the previously established front guide straight up from the top of the head at a 90-degree elevation.

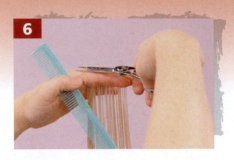

6 Cut horizontally.

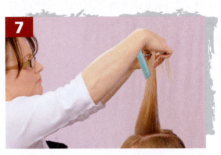

7 Use this section as a traveling guide. Pick up a small portion of it with each newly parted section and cut horizontally, moving back toward the crown. Continue to use the same holding position of 90-degree elevation (straight up from the top of the head) and horizontal cutting position throughout.

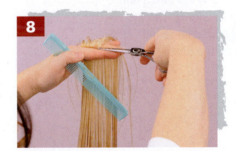

8 Cross-check your work through this top area by taking vertical sections and holding them straight up from the top of the head. Clean up any unevenness.

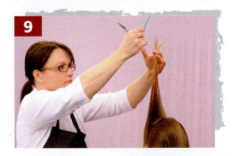

9 Move to the crest area. Part off a vertical section at the front hairline. Direct this section up and out from the crest area and cut with your fingers in the position shown. This connects to the length from the top.

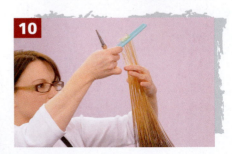

10 Use the first section as a traveling guide to cut the sections behind it. Angle the fingers diagonally and continue cutting outward.

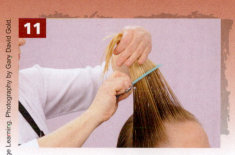

11 Take pie-shaped partings from the crown as you move from the side toward the center back, cutting to the established guideline.

12 Repeat the steps on the left side, starting with the establishment of the traveling guide.

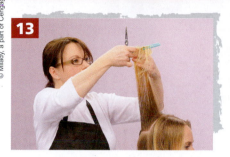

13 Work toward the back of the head and use pie-shaped partings as you cut the crown and nape. Continue until you reach the center back. Move to the right side and complete in the same manner.

14 In this technique you are cutting toward the perimeter. Continue this technique to the center back as a control measure for blending all lengths outward.

15 Finish the design by separating the textured hair with the tips of your fingers.

Create

Apply this technique to different hair lengths, colors, and textures for almost endless possibilities.

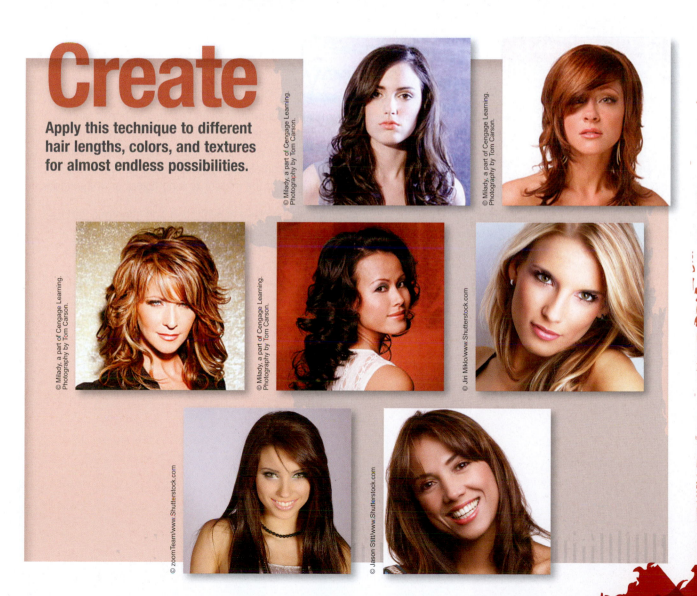

Part 3: The Layered Haircut

49

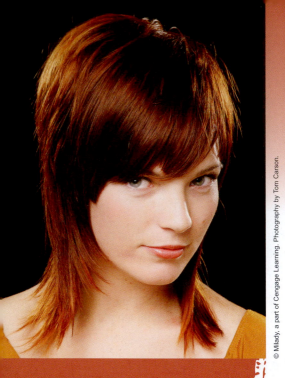

Heavy Layers Haircut on Short Hair— Full Layers

Implements and Materials

You will need all of the following implements, materials, and supplies:

- **Cutting cape**
- **Cutting or styling comb**
- **Haircutting shears**
- **Neck strip**
- **Sectioning clips**
- **Spray bottle with water**
- **Towels**
- **Wide-tooth comb**

Overview

In this shape the entire haircut is progressively layered—shorter lengths in the interior work toward longer lengths around the perimeter. It is very important to consider the hair density as it will determine the final look of this cut. Shown here is the completely layered shape. Lengths move progressively from short layers in the interior to long layers on the exterior.

These technical steps follow the client consultation and shampoo service.

Technical Drawing

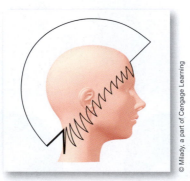

Procedure

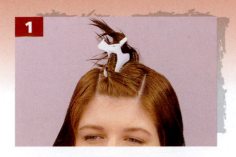

1 Comb and detangle the hair. Part out a rectangular section from the front hairline to the crown and from the center of the eye on either side.

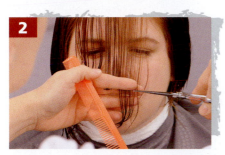

2 Take a ½-inch (1.25 cm) section from the front (at the hairline), comb it down the front of the face and holding it at as close to a 0-degree elevation as possible, cut it horizontally at the tip of the nose.

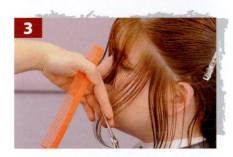

3 Next, take a ½-inch (1.25 cm) section along the side, from the fringe section at the top to the temple area. Hold the hair in the natural falling position, connect and blend into the fringe length previously cut. Repeat on the opposite side and check the lengths for balance.

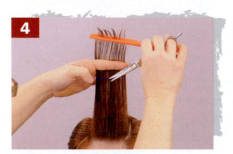

4 Starting at the front of the rectangular parting, release and cut horizontal sections through the top section. Use the initially cut section to establish the traveling guide. Each section is held 90-degrees straight out from the curve of the head and cut horizontally.

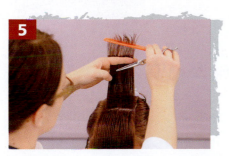

5 Work all the way back to the crown, picking up a portion of the previously cut section each time to act as a traveling guide. Comb and distribute the hair neatly out from the head and cut horizontally. Check lines for evenness.

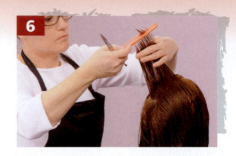

6   Having completed the top area, part out vertical sections through the crest area for layering through this panel. Direct the lengths straight up and out from the head and begin cutting out toward the perimeter area using a traveling guide.

7   Continue this holding and cutting position to the center back. The partings are pie-shaped around the crown area.

8   Move to the next panel. Part off vertically, holding the hair straight, and begin cutting to blend to the perimeter frame.

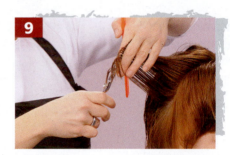

9   Using this section as a traveling guide, work toward the left side, cutting the side panels. The panels should be about 2-inches (5 cm) wide. Work toward the nape with these vertical sections.

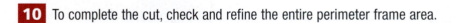

10   To complete the cut, check and refine the entire perimeter frame area.

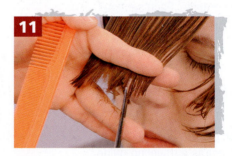

11   Detail the front perimeter to suit the face. Here, point cutting softens the look. Place the fingers according to the depth of point cutting that will be made into the ends of the hair. Observe and check the softness as it is developing.

12   The layered cut gives the hair a lot of movement. The finished style shows the cut with a subtle flip in the nape area. This shape offers a variety of styling options.

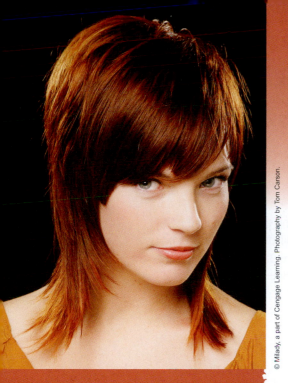

© Milady, a part of Cengage Learning. Photography by Tom Carson.

Heavy Layers Haircut on Short Hair—Full Layers Finishing Option

Implements and Materials

You will need all of the following implements, materials, and supplies:

- **Shampoo cape**
- **Neck strip**
- **Sectioning clips**
- **Spray bottle with water**
- **Towels**
- **Wide-tooth comb**
- **Heat-resistant rubber-based half-round brush**
- **Blowdryer**
- **Blowdryer nozzle**
- **Blowdryer diffuser**
- **Appropriate styling products**

Overview

Here is another example of styling the hair to conform to the contours of its shape. The finished style highlights the shape of the cut, and the drying technique you use accentuates the layering above the ears and through the top of the head.

These technical steps follow the client consultation, shampoo service, and haircut.

Procedure

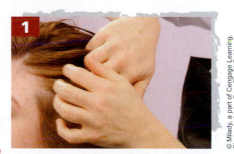

© Milady, a part of Cengage Learning. Photography by Gary David Gold.

1 Apply a styling product of your choice and work it through the hair.

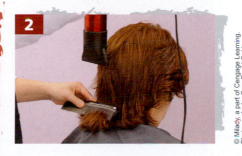

© Milady, a part of Cengage Learning. Photography by Gary David Gold.

2 Holding the hair very close around the perimeter shape with a comb, dry the hair, following the comb with the blowdryer. This will keep this area closely contoured.

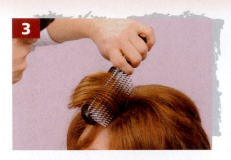

3 Move to the fringe area next. Using a rubber-based half-round blowdrying brush, smooth the hair by rolling the brush under as you dry. Note how flat the base area is held when turning the ends back and toward the side.

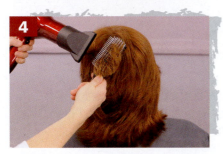

4 Continue into the crown area.

5 Comb through the nape area if it needs lift.

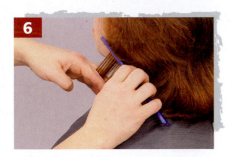

6 Blend and connect the side sections with the front.

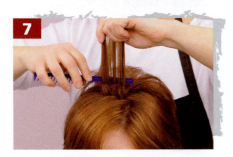

7 Use a teasing comb to separate and detail the lengths. Backcomb the crown area, then detail, using your comb and fingers.

8 Continue detailing. This is where your artistry is expressed.

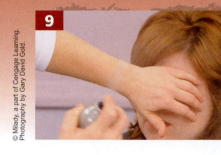

9

9 Detail the edges. Spray for the desired hold.

10 The finished style shows closely contoured layers through the exterior with an emphasis on directional volume through the fringe and crown areas.

Create

Apply this technique to different hair lengths, colors, and textures for almost endless possibilities.

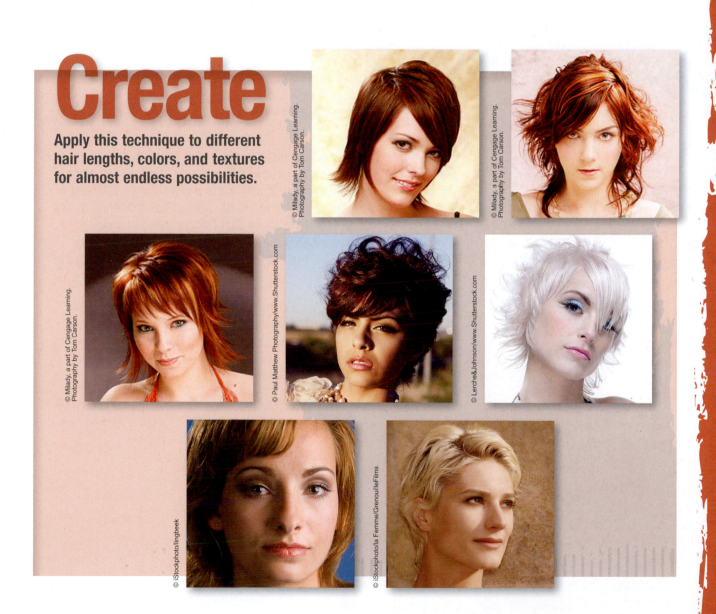

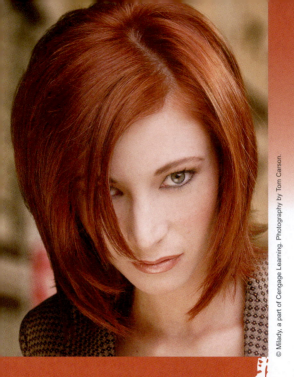
© Milady, a part of Cengage Learning. Photography by Tom Carson.

Layered Square Shape Haircut

Implements and Materials

You will need all of the following implements, materials, and supplies:

- **Cutting cape**
- **Cutting or styling comb**
- **Haircutting shears**
- **Neck strip**
- **Sectioning clips**
- **Spray bottle with water**
- **Towels**
- **Wide-tooth comb**

Overview

This dynamic short shape will provide your client with a silhouette that features weight emphasis and length to frame the face and add volume to the back of the head. The shape is more closely contoured or layered above the ears and through the top area of the head. It is a very wearable, distinctive geometric shape that can be styled in a variety of ways—ideal for the client who likes to wear her hair short or for the client who may have a less-than-perfect head shape. You will revisit this cut again and again.

When performing this cut on a client in its entirety, you will first cut the perimeter frame along the desired lines either as a blunt or graduated shape. Shown here is the finished layered shape. The weight areas within this haircut emphasize a unique dimension. This haircut is suitable for a wide range of clients.

These technical steps follow the client consultation and shampoo service.

Technical Drawing

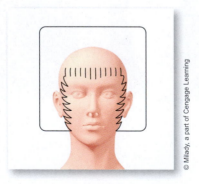

© Milady, a part of Cengage Learning

Procedure

1 First, comb the hair in natural fall and establish a center part.

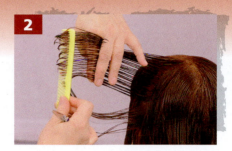

2 Part out a ½-inch (1.25 cm) vertical section from behind the ear to establish a guide. Considering desired finished length, texture, and head shape, determine the length of your guide. Comb this hair straight out from the side of the head (into a horizontal holding position) and cut this section along a vertical line.

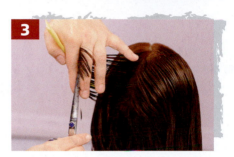

3 Bring the front area, in ½-inch (1.25 cm) sections, back to this guide. Notice that while you are holding the hair straight out from the side, the cutting position is vertical. Note also that the scissor position is vertical.

4 Bring sections from the back forward to this guide and cut using ½-inch (1.25 cm) sections. Work all the way to the center back with pie-shaped sections around the crown.

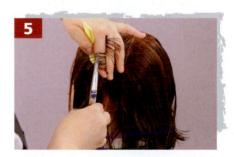

5 Repeat the procedure outlined until you reach the center of the back of the head.

6 Take a ½-inch (1.25 cm) vertical section from directly behind the ear and cut to the guide.

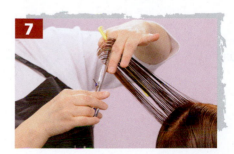

7 Using wedge-shaped partings, bring sections from the back forward, toward the side guide, and cut. Work all the way to the center back.

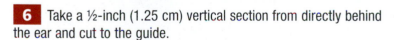

8 In preparation for cutting the nape, take a ½-inch (1.25 cm) vertical section from the occipital bone to the nape. Hold it straight out from the curve of the head, and cut it vertically.

9 Bring the hair from both the left and right of the nape-section stationery guide and cut. Again, use ½-inch (1.25 cm) sections and direct the hair back to your stationery guide until you run out of length toward the ears.

10 Complete the right side of the head in the same manner.

11 Establish a guide for cutting the top, front, and crown areas.

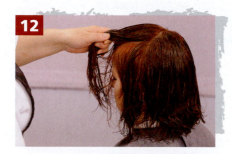

12 Part off a section on the top of the head from the hairline to the crown and from the middle of the eye to the middle of the eye.

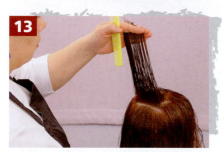

13 Part a ½-inch (1.25 cm) horizontal section across the top of the head. Comb and hold this section straight up, then cut it horizontally to establish your length guide.

14 Bring all the hair in front of this section back to the guide and cut working toward the front hairline.

15 Part from the top of the ear and cut the guideline to blend with the previously cut hair at the top of the head. Bring the crown sections forward to the stationery guide and cut.

16 Use ½-inch (1.25 cm) sections for control and cut until you no longer have enough length to reach the guide.

17 Next, part down the middle of the head. Then, on the left side, use the top and side guide to cut the hair over the ear. Cut at a 90-degree elevation. Move to the right side and do the same.

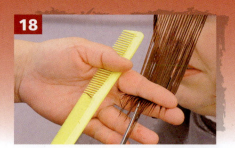

18 Part off the fringe to cut the front perimeter into the desired shape.

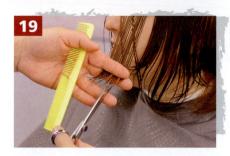

19 Use a point cutting technique to define and create a softened edge.

20 The layering technique used in this haircut has created weight corners. These weight corners may be softened by holding the hair straight out from the curve of the head and point cutting into the lengths to diffuse the edge.

21 Use the point cutting technique in front of and over the ear, holding the hair with the comb.

22 To complete the cut, refine the side edges. Strive for a soft, wispy effect using variations on the point cutting technique.

23 The finished style has dynamic movement and texture with a shape that allows for easily created volume and dimension.

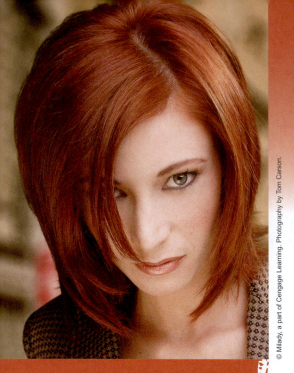

Layered Square Shape Haircut Finishing Option

Implements and Materials

You will need all of the following implements, materials, and supplies:

- **Shampoo cape**
- **Neck strip**
- **Sectioning clips**
- **Spray bottle with water**
- **Towels**
- **Wide-tooth comb**
- **Heat-resistant rubber-based brush**
- **Blowdryer**
- **Blowdryer nozzle**
- **Blowdryer diffuser**
- **Appropriate styling products**

Overview

The styling of shorter shapes is usually dictated by the way in which the hair was cut. Clients choose shorter shapes because they want ease of handling—so the finish should be easy care, too.

These technical steps follow the client consultation, shampoo service, and haircut.

Procedure

1 Begin by applying foam to the crown area. Work the product through the hair.

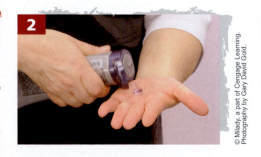

2 Next, apply a styling product of your choice. For our finishing option, we are using a liquid gel for sleek control.

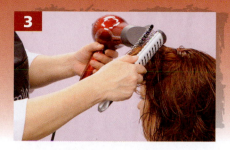

3 Begin to dry the front area. Direct the lengths and the airflow into the desired movement. The airflow is directed along the top surface. A vent brush facilitates even, thorough airflow.

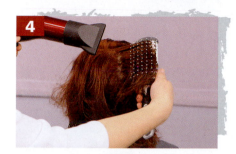

4 Work around the crown.

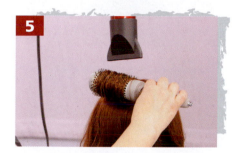

5 Switch to a round brush and continue to work in the crown area. The goal is to maximize volume in this area.

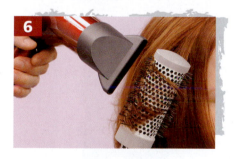

6 Continue through to the side section on either side, connecting with the directional placement in the crown.

7 Comb the hair with a wide-tooth comb.

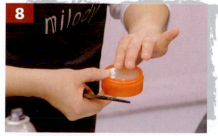

8 Detail the ends with your fingers, using a small amount of spray or pomade on the fingertips.

Part 3: The Layered Haircut

Layered Square Shape Haircut
Finishing Option continued

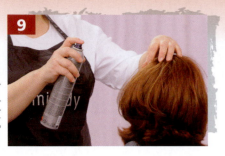

9 Spray to finish. Lift for volume in the crown—balance the shape while spraying.

10 Use your creative artistry to finish this design. Directional movement, volume, and enhanced texture are all features of this finished style.

Create

Apply this technique to different hair lengths, colors, and textures for almost endless possibilities.

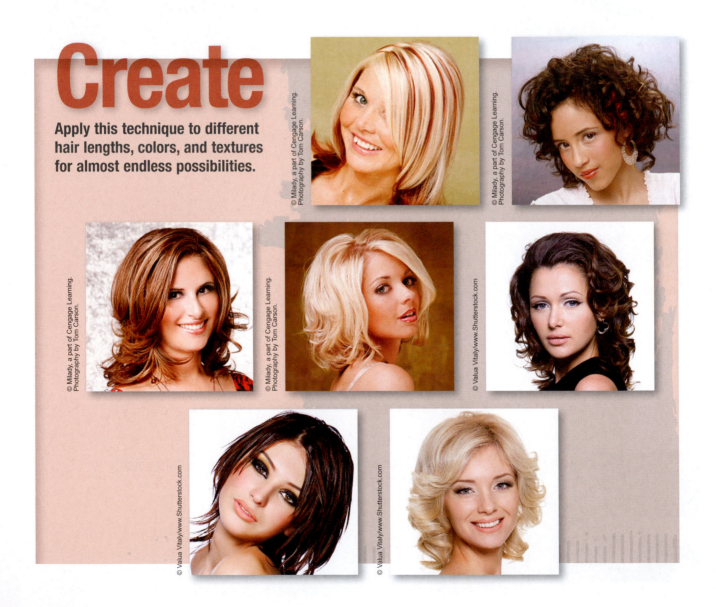

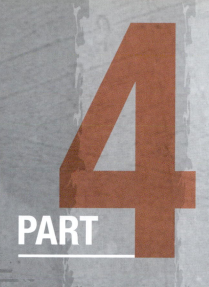

PART 4

Technical Options For Consideration

Considering that no two heads of hair are exactly the same due to hair texture, density, and growth patterns, it is easy to understand why no one tool, technique, or procedure will give identical results. Selecting the best tools and techniques for the desired haircut can be equally as important as choosing the hair design for the client.

From humanity's beginning, there has always been a need to cut hair. In early times, sharpened edges honed from stone, bone, and shell formed the tools for cutting and shaving—for example, Egyptian royalty shaved their heads and wore wigs. Ancient Greek sculpture and artifacts portray men with hairstyles that would have required cutting. Images of haircuts are found in early dynasty drawings from Asia.

Through time, the concept of haircutting (or not cutting the hair) has been a sign of a person's marital, religious, and social status. Interestingly enough, religious beliefs can sometimes dictate the cutting of hair today, just as in the past. Ceremonial tools have also been created for the cutting of hair.

With the discovery of metal working, man fashioned blades of iron, bronze, silver, and gold—sometimes ornate and jewel encrusted. A single blade or razor was the only choice for haircutting until the invention of two blades or razors that were hinged to form the first shears. Credit for this discovery has been given to shepherds in need of a better tool for the harvesting of wool.

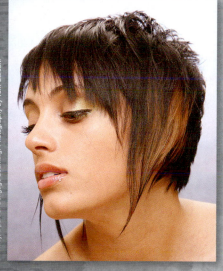

The electric hair clipper, with either single or multiple moving blades, was first developed for livestock and then later applied for use on humans. In modern medical technology, surgical cutting is often done with a laser. Is laser the next tool in the hairdresser's arsenal? Only time, technology, and your needs as hairdressers will tell!

Wet Hair versus Dry Hair

A consideration before beginning any haircut is the amount of moisture in the hair, or to put it simply: how wet or dry the hair is and why? Cutting damp hair that has been freshly shampooed would seem the logical sequence in a haircut, but many hairstylists will list a number of exceptions for cutting hair that is damp.

One reason for cutting hair when it is dry is to compensate for the effect of growth patterns and hair texture on the finished style. Another consideration, and the one with the most differing opinions, regards the cutting of textured or curly hair. One school of thought is to have the curly hair in its natural dry state and to separate and cut each ringlet individually. This can be a very time consuming yet effective process, and it is often desired by the curly haired client who embraces her natural hair texture. The opposite approach is to have curly or textured hair dried straight in preparation for a precision cut. This can be a very successful technique for the client who will wear his or her hair straightened chemically or straightened temporarily through applied heat. The most frequently used technique is neither wet nor dry cutting, but a combination of the two.

Many stylists will begin a cut on wet hair and detail or finish on dry hair; they will also often precut on dry hair to establish guidelines and then complete the cut on wet hair. Some stylists will sometimes, unfortunately, make this decision depending on the time scheduled or by habit instead of by what will give the best results for the client. It is your responsibility as a professional to make the best possible decision based on your experience. Try wet, dry, or any combination on as many differing hair textures as possible to help you in learning to make the best choice in each situation for each client.

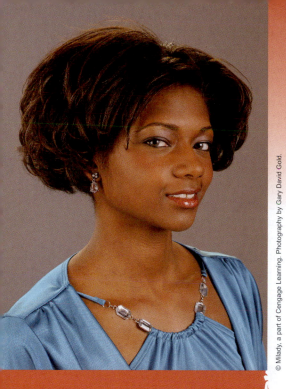

Blunt Haircut on Dry Hair

Overview

Time management is a top priority with today's hectic pace of living. A good time-management technique you can use for your clients with very curly hair is to invest more time in chemical relaxer services, conditioning treatments, and preparation of the hair by blowdrying smooth (pre-prep) before you begin cutting and finishing.

Hair that is highly textured (curly, for instance) appears completely different when wet. When this type of hair dries, it contracts in length as the curl pulls it up. Cutting hair of this type when it's dry gives you more control over the creation of the shape. Once the hair is relaxed to be straight and smooth, an unlimited variety of sculpted styles can be created from this foundation.

The dry-cutting technique is a classic, condensed cutting and finishing concept. Preexisting internal layers flow over the perimeter blunt weight line. The notched areas around the front hairline are cut bluntly.

These technical steps follow the client consultation and shampoo service. The following technical steps will be completed after the client consultation, the relaxer treatment, and the conditioning and color treatments. Once these are completed, blowdry the hair smooth.

Implements and Materials

You will need all of the following implements, materials, and supplies:

- **Cutting cape**
- **Cutting or styling comb**
- **Haircutting shears**
- **Neck strip**
- **Sectioning clips**
- **Spray bottle with water**
- **Towels**
- **Wide-tooth comb**

Technical Drawing

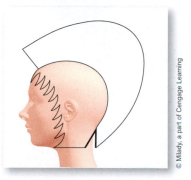

Blunt Haircut on Dry Hair continued
Procedure

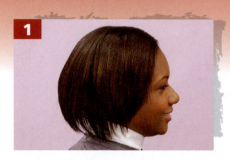

1 After blowdrying, use a dry-wrapping technique to straighten, control, and smooth the hair for dry cutting. Brush or comb all the dry hair around the head, then blowdry again for a few minutes or put under a warm dryer to "set" the wrapped hair direction. This will create natural-looking curved movement, with the hair contouring close to the head shape, a result that is not generally achieved by chemically relaxing, blowdrying, or ironing hair.

2 Now the hair is ready for a dry designer cut. Comb the hair in the direction of the desired cut using a side part

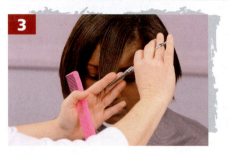

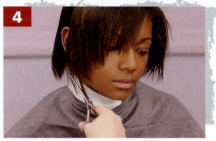

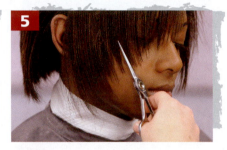

3 Diagonally blunt cut a line over the left eye. Part the hair across the head from ear to ear and comb the hair in the back away.

4 After completing the fringe area, move to the right side. Cut your guideline and notch cut into it.

5 Keep in mind that this technique is free-form in nature—meaning that you are notching into the lengths around the front hairline at measured, slightly irregular intervals. Continue to create your design around the face using the notch cutting technique.

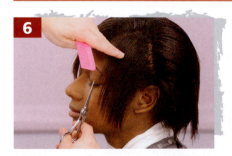

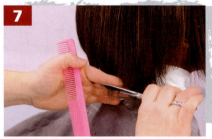

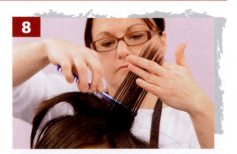

6 After completing the right side, move to the left side. Continue to create your design around the face using the notch cutting technique.

7 After completing the left and right sides, move to the back section. Create a blunt weight line at the desired length. Check the line for balance.

8 Backcomb the hair on the top of the head to create a base for volume through the crown area. Use hair spray on the backcombed areas for added support. Smooth the backcombed hair into place. The result is an entire head of hair that is consistent in texture, with smooth soft movement.

Part 4: Technical Options For Consideration

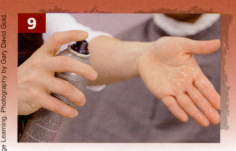

9 Spray the hair for hold. Spray some hair spray on your fingers and detail around the face.

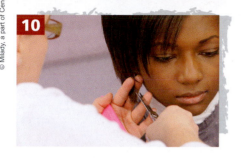

10 The client's makeover is complete. Her hair has been transformed!

11 The consistent texture and soft movement complement the closely contoured blunt shape, results that are accentuated through the dry-wrapping and dry-haircutting techniques. The finished style is progressive but classic, with hair that is shiny and silky.

Create

Apply this technique to different hair lengths, colors, and textures for almost endless possibilities.

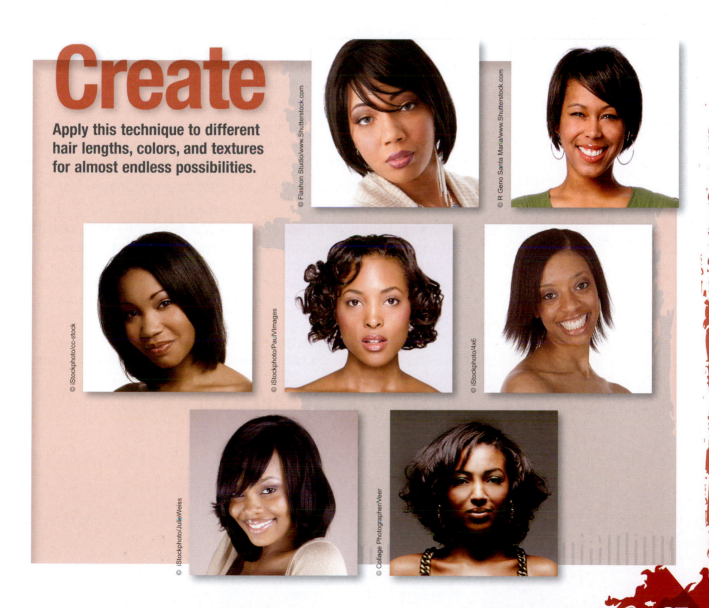

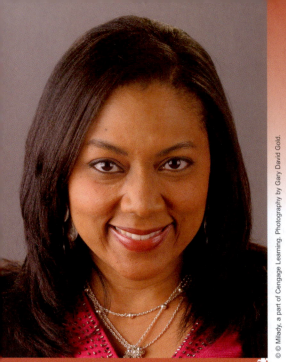

Heavy Layers Haircut on Pressed Hair

Implements and Materials

You will need all of the following implements, materials, and supplies:

- **Cutting cape**
- **Cutting or styling comb**
- **Haircutting shears**
- **Neck strip**
- **Sectioning clips**
- **Spray bottle with water**
- **Towels**
- **Wide-tooth comb**

Overview

A client who prefers to wear her curly hair in a smooth and straight finished style has two choices—she can either chemically relax her hair or press the natural curl into a smooth texture. If the client chooses the nonchemical pressing alternative, you must first press the hair smooth and then cut it dry. This will ensure the creation of the most accurate, precise shape.

Techniques for straightening hair have come and gone through the years, but applying heat to dry, curly hair along with pressure is a method that has endured. Pressing hair to straighten it will always be a popular technique, and it is important to know the proper method for cutting a pressed head of hair.

Heavy layers flow through the interior and along the perimeter frame that has been cut blunt.

While many haircuts are performed on damp hair, hair that has been pressed will need to be cut when it is dry. Not only does the dry method maintain the straightening achieved by pressing, but it also permits greater precision in creating the shape because you can perfectly predict where the hair will fall in the finished style. Whether dried straight and smooth or dried naturally, a precise shape is ensured.

Before beginning this service, blowdry the hair and press it with a pressing iron. After you complete the cut, curl the hair to add soft movement and body.

Technical Drawing

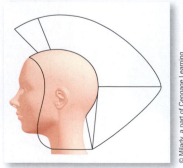

Procedure

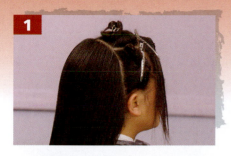

1 Begin by dividing the hair into five sections: fringe area, crown, right side, left side, and back. Comb the entire back section into its natural falling position and create your guide, beginning in the center back, and cut toward the left side—hold the hair straight down and cut a horizontal line using a low, one-finger elevation.

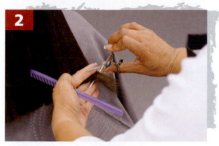

2 Complete the right side in the same manner.

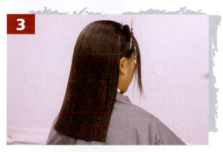

3 Release the hair in the crown area. Notice that the previously cut layers do not reach the blunt perimeter. These lengths will get cut during the layering process.

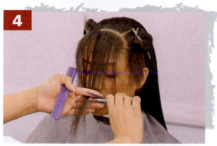

4 At the front of the head, comb the fringe section forward and, using the tip of the nose as a guide, cut straight across and adjacent to the outside corner of the eye. Repeat the cut on the other half of the fringe.

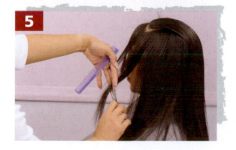

5 Move to the left side of the head. Comb the side and top sections slightly forward and, using the front fringe area as a guide, cut the side diagonally from the nose down to the side guide, blending the fringe and side areas and framing the face.

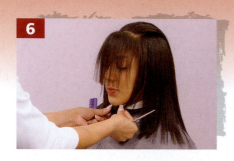

6 Move to the right side and continue framing the face, blending the hair at a diagonal with the fringe area. Check sides for balance.

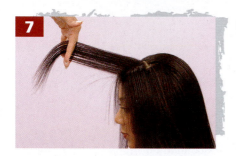

7 Move to the top front area. Part out a triangular-shaped section from the top center crown to the front hairline.

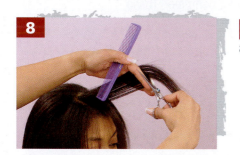

8 Hold the hair straight out from the top to the front guideline and begin cutting along the fingers to create a length increase.

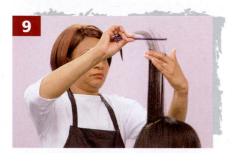

9 Move around the head. Continue to make pie-shaped partings around the crown, holding them at a 90-degree angle from the side of the head and cutting out to the traveling guide that you have created.

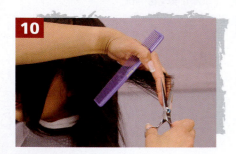

10 Move through the crown of the head. Hold the hair at a 90-degree angle from the curve of the head and cut. Once the cut is completed, add some curl to the finished style. The completed style has fluid movement and frames the face with a soft fringe.

Part 4: Technical Options For Consideration

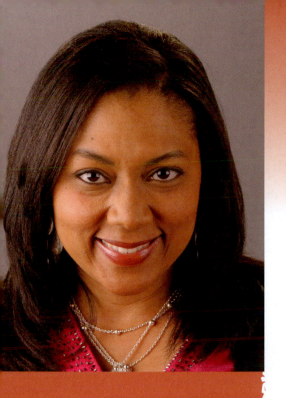

Flat Iron and Curl on Heavy Layers Finishing Option

Implements and Materials

You will need all of the following implements, materials, and supplies:

- **Shampoo cape**
- **Neck strip**
- **Sectioning clips**
- **Spray bottle with water**
- **Towels**
- **Wide-tooth comb**
- **Heat-resistant rubber-based brush**
- **Electric or thermal pressing comb**
- **Curling iron**
- **Blowdryer**
- **Blowdryer nozzle**
- **Blowdryer diffuser**
- **Appropriate styling products**

Overview

A press and curl is a temporary thermal-straightening technique used on very curly hair; the hair will revert to its natural state when shampooed. It may also be affected by perspiration, humidity, or other elements. No chemicals are used in this service—some clients do not want chemicals in their hair. If they are on medication, pregnant, or have extremely dry scalps, clients will want a press and curl because it is chemical-free.

These technical steps follow the client consultation, shampoo service, and towel-drying the hair.

Procedure

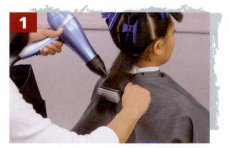

1 Divide the head into four sections. Beginning at the back, left side, blowdry the hair using a blowdryer with nozzle and a hard-rubber brush to heat and straighten the hair. Work section by section to dry the hair.

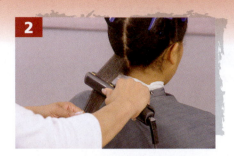

2 Once the hair is completely dried, divide it again into four sections. Before beginning, be sure to test the heat of your flat iron before placing it on the hair.

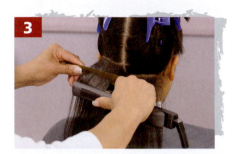

3 Next, beginning on the back left side, take a 1½-inch (3.75 cm) horizontal subsection. Then, while holding the hair firmly in one hand and the flat iron in the other, apply the flat iron to the hair as close to the scalp as possible and slide the iron along the length of the hair, to the ends.

4 Now, move to the right side and take a 1½-inch (3.75 cm) horizontal subsection and flat iron this section in the same manner. Continue to flat iron the hair throughout the entire back sections.

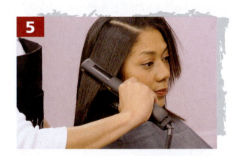

5 When you have finished the entire back, move to the right side and begin flat ironing in the same manner. Hold the hair with a gentle but firm tension as you glide the flat iron along the hair.

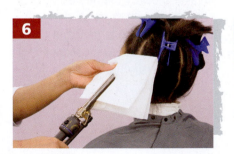

6 Move to the left side and flat iron the hair in the same manner. Once all of the hair has been flat ironed you will need to divide the hair into four sections again to begin curling the hair with a curling iron. Before putting the curling iron into the hair, test the heat of the iron by placing it on a white paper towel. Adjust the temperature of the iron if needed.

© Milady, a part of Cengage Learning. Photography by Gary David Gold.

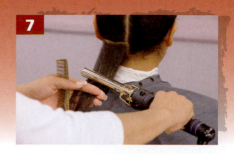

7 Beginning in the nape, take a 1½-inch (3.75 cm) section and test your curling iron by placing it on top of the section. Slide the iron down the hair shaft while firmly holding the hair—this is called *silking* the hair. Remember to always leave the curling iron slightly open until you get to the end of the hair.

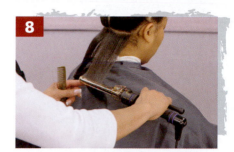

8 When you get to the ends of the hair, close the curling iron and work the ends of the hair into the middle of the curl.

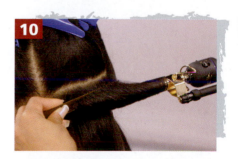

9 Place a hard-rubber comb under the curling iron and roll the curling iron to the scalp.

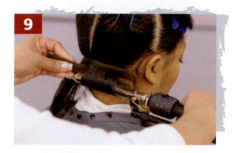

10 Hold the curling iron in the hair until you can no longer see the ends of the hair. Slide the iron out of the curl.

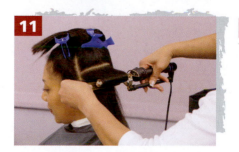

11 Continue to curl the hair in this manner working upward toward the crown.

Flat Iron and Curl on Heavy Layers
Finishing Option continued

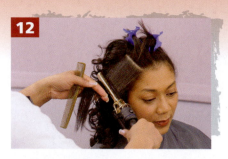

12 Once the back sections are curled, move to the side and begin curling the hair using the feed-in method.

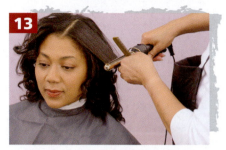

13 Complete the other side in this manner.

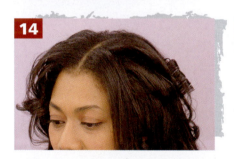

14 When the flat ironing and curl is completed and ready to be styled, notice the smooth lines of the curls.

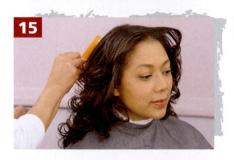

15 Using a rake-type styling comb, comb the hair toward the back of the head to smooth and accentuate the curls you have made.

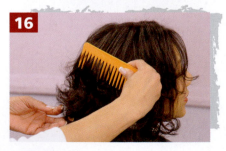

16 As you reach the center back of the head, in addition to using your rake, use your fingers to isolate strands of curls. Highlighting curls at different lengths will also make the layers in the haircut easier to see.

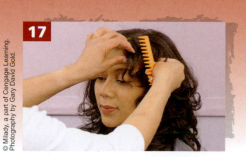

17

17 Repeat on the left side, pulling out pieces of hair to softly frame the face. Detail the surface for the desired textural movement.

18 Using a flat iron to straighten and a curling iron to create uniform sized curls creates a softened shape with textural and directional movement and dimension.

Create

Apply this technique to different hair lengths, colors, and textures for almost endless possibilities.

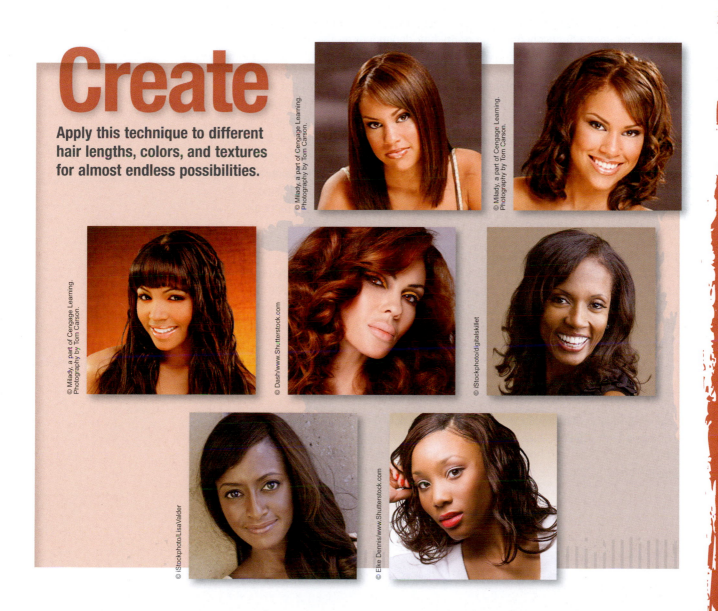

Shears, Razors, or Clippers—Which to Choose

How do you choose between using shears, razors, or clippers for creating an incredible haircut? To make the right choice of a tool or tools requires an understanding of the function, the unique characteristics, and the results of each of these tools.

The shear will probably be the most frequently used tool in your career. Shears are mainly used to cut blunt or straight lines in hair. They can also be used for many texturizing techniques such as point cutting, slide cutting, and notching. When you work with shears, the ends are cut blunt. This is why many stylists will choose shears when cutting curly or coarse hair, and when precision cutting is desired. A shear can be used effectively on damp or dry hair dependent on the hair type, texture, and result desired.

Razors are mainly used when a softer effect on the ends of the hair is desired. When working with a razor, the ends are cut at an angle, and the line is not blunt. This produces softer shapes with a more visible separation, or a feathered effect on the ends. Any haircut you can create with shears can also be accomplished with a razor, but the razor cut will deliver different results. With a razor there is always some degree of tension on the hair. Tension is a consideration on hair with texture, irregular growth patterns, and hair that is too short to hold for cutting. When using a razor, the hair must remain damp while cutting or it may cause frizziness, damage, or possibly some discomfort to the client.

Clippers are similar to shears in the ability to cut without any tension as in the shear-over-comb or clipper-over-comb techniques. Even though most haircuts you create with shears can be duplicated with a clipper, many clients may be uncomfortable with a haircut completed exclusively with a clipper. Clippers work best on barely damp-to-dry hair, making clippers a great choice for cross-checking shorter haircuts, blunt haircuts, and cuts on extremely textured/curly hair.

On damaged or overprocessed hair, avoid using the razor and be sure to cut with little or no tension.

The above are just a few guidelines concerning the selection of tools for a haircut and do not replace what is learned from the experience of working with the different tools. Knowing how to choose the right tool for each unique cutting application gives a stylist the opportunity for endless creativity in haircutting.

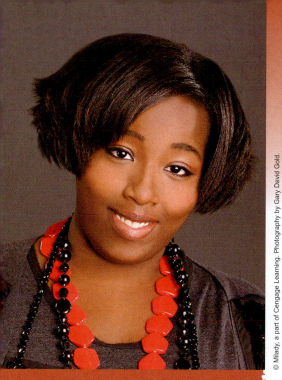

© Milady, a part of Cengage Learning. Photography by Gary David Gold.

Layered Graduation Haircut with Clippers

Implements and Materials

You will need all of the following implements, materials, and supplies:

- **Cutting cape**
- **Cutting or styling comb**
- **Clipper**
- **Neck strip**
- **Sectioning clips**
- **Spray bottle with water**
- **Towels**
- **Wide-tooth comb**

Overview

Clipper cutting decreases cutting time—which means faster service. Using this free-form method will give you accurate results because the clipper offers precision in creating lines. Generally, when you use a clipper, the emphasis of the cut will be on the silhouette.

For extra control, some stylists use both hands to hold the clipper. If you are holding the clipper with one hand and the hair or a comb with the other, remember that the more tension you use, the more precise the line your clipper will create. Before you begin any cut with your clipper, however, you must envision where you are going with it. In this design, interior layers flow over the perimeter graduation. A blunt fringe adds dramatic flair. Precise lines are easily created using the clipper cutting technique.

Technical Drawing

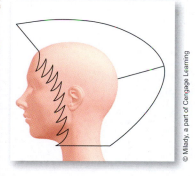

© Milady, a part of Cengage Learning

Layered Graduation Haircut with Clippers continued

Procedure

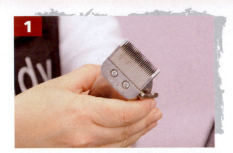

1 Before beginning, examine the clipper blade to ensure that it is in top-notch condition. Clean and oil the clipper regularly.

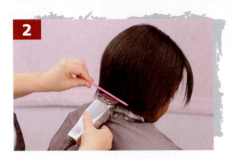

2 Establish the perimeter guide at the back of the head, in the nape area. Point the clipper blade toward the neck and use the clipper to create the line from ear to ear. Work methodically with the blade inverted against the hair as shown.

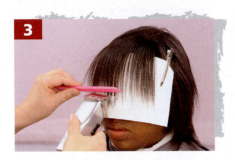

3 At the front of the head, section off the fringe area. For instructional purposes only, a piece of white cardboard has been clipped under the fringe. Cut first at the center of the fringe section, then cut the line outward on either side to the outside corners of the eyes. Leave the fringe slightly longer if you intend to use an iron, as this will make the fringe look shorter.

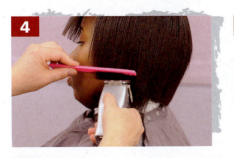

4 Move to the left side. Establish a new length for the side. This design length does not connect to the back section. From the tip of the earlobe to the jawline is the ideal length on the appropriate head shape. Note the new position of the clipper; it is used in this manner to sweep the blade sideways along the line. Cut to refine.

5 Create the same perimeter line on the right side. If cutting away from the head, hold the hair between the fingers.

6 Using your mirror and standing directly behind the client's head, check for balance in the length of your cut.

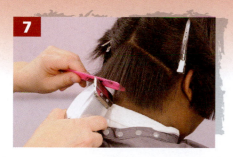

7 Section the back to begin tapering the neckline area. Hold a section of hair straight out from the curve of the head with the comb angled as shown. Establish your first cut with the clipper. Remember to envision where you are going with the cut.

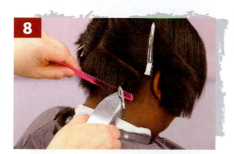

8 Continue to create graduation toward the outer edges of the nape, using the clipper-over-comb technique. As you work toward the occipital bone, allow your elevation to increase gradually as you move outward from the neckline.

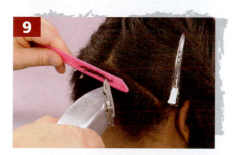

9 Hold the comb so that it is closer to the head along the back edge of the comb and farther away from the head along its teeth. Note the high graduation developing through this area.

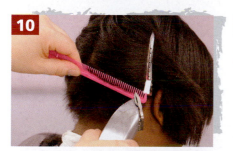

10 Consistency in angling the comb, hair length, and graduation is essential. Blend from the center area toward the area behind the ear.

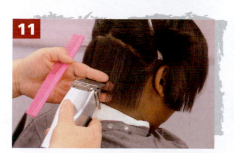

11 Control the hair lengths by holding them between your fingers and cutting against the fingers. When you are cutting, blend the remainder of the back to the graduated nape area and into the sides.

12 Once the entire back section is cut, refine the sculptured shape for softness and precision using the clipper.

Layered Graduation Haircut with Clippers
continued

© Milady, a part of Cengage Learning. Photography by Gary David Gold.

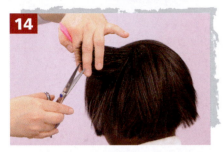

13 Through the top of the head, you will use a condensed cutting technique with large sections that radiate around the curve of the head. Comb a large section at a 90-degree angle from behind the fringe. Begin cutting out from the fringe to the crown lengths. You will use this as a guide to move around the head with radial sections.

14 Comb and check the cut around the entire perimeter of the head for detail, trimming any uneven hair.

15 The finished style is smooth and voluminous, with graduation creating body at the nape.

Create

Apply this technique to different hair lengths, colors, and textures for almost endless possibilities.

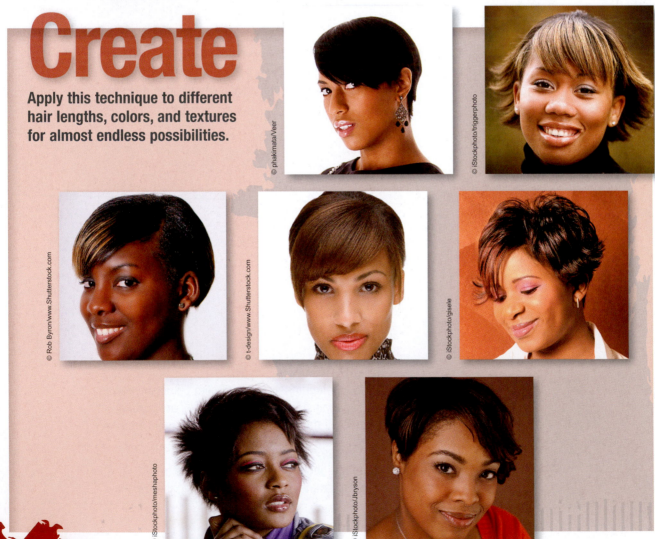

© phakimata/Veer

© iStockphoto/triggerphoto

© Rob Byron/www.Shutterstock.com

© t-design/www.Shutterstock.com

© iStockphoto/gisele

© iStockphoto/meshaphoto

© iStockphoto/Jbryson

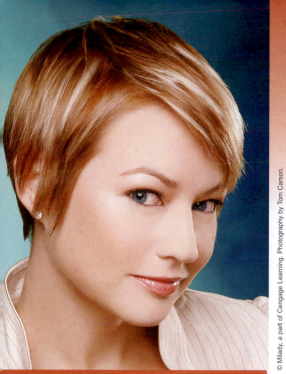

© Milady, a part of Cengage Learning. Photography by Tom Carson.

Layered Razor Haircut

Implements and Materials

You will need all of the following implements, materials, and supplies:

- **Cutting cape**
- **Cutting or styling comb**
- **Razor**
- **Neck strip**
- **Sectioning clips**
- **Spray bottle with water**
- **Towels**
- **Wide-tooth comb**

Overview

The razor is a superb tool for making the hair fluid with movement. Razor cutting tapers the lengths, creating a variety of lengths and eliminating any angularity. This type of cutting is used whenever a soft, diffused, wispy, or fringed edge is desired. Using the razor requires a light versus a heavy-handed approach. In this cut, the razor is used to create softly variegated texture along the edges as opposed to the blunt straight edge achieved with the shear.

The heavily layered shape will be very light and airy—rounded throughout the interior and contoured close through the nape.

Technical Drawing

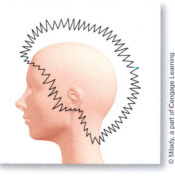

Layered Razor Haircut continued

Procedure

1 Comb all the hair back off of the face. Beginning on the left side, take a ½-inch (1.25 cm) section along the front hairline. Comb it against the face. Holding the hair in a low elevation, position the razor guard toward you and the blade against the hair.

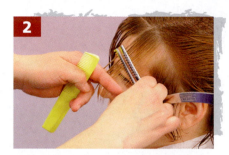

2 Place the razor at that point along the strand where you want to begin to cut. Move or etch the razor back and forth along the strand as shown.

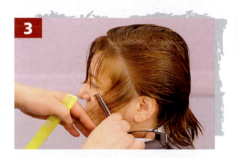

3 Cut parallel to the hairline using the razor to create a taper. Complete cutting the left side in this manner.

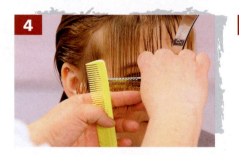

4 Move to the right side and repeat.

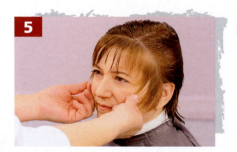

5 Check both sides for balance.

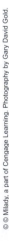

Part 4: Technical Options For Consideration

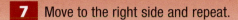

6 Beginning on the left side, using the previously cut hairline perimeter guide as your traveling guides, work from the front to the back, razor cutting the hair in ½-inch (1.25 cm) sections. Do not cut any lower than the occipital bone.

7 Move to the right side and repeat.

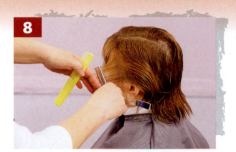

8 To blend the top and sides, take ½-inch (1.25 cm) sections across the top and, using the previously cut side as your guide, use the razor to notch cut the ends. Etch along the top of the hair to taper from the mid-shaft toward the ends, removing the length just above the fingers.

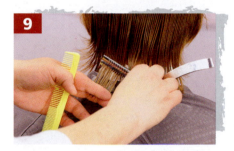

9 Move to the back and taper the nape. Hold the sections slightly outward at a 30- to 45-degree angle, then etch along the top surface to create the desired length.

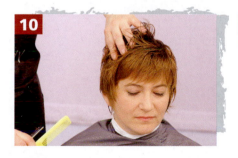

10 The variety of lengths throughout the silhouette creates volume without any hard edges.

11 Leave the hair fringed and soft or cut the hair short to contrast with the longer frame around the face.

12 The finished style is softly tapered throughout for movement and dimension.

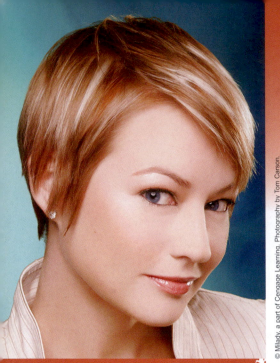

Layered Razor Haircut Finishing Option

© Milady, a part of Cengage Learning. Photography by Tom Carson.

Implements and Materials

You will need all of the following implements, materials, and supplies:

- **Shampoo cape**
- **Neck strip**
- **Sectioning clips**
- **Spray bottle with water**
- **Towels**
- **Wide-tooth comb**
- **Heat-resistant rubber-based paddle brush**
- **Blowdryer**
- **Blowdryer nozzle**
- **Blowdryer diffuser**
- **Appropriate styling products**

Overview

Razor cutting provides a wide range of opportunity for you to express your artistic and professional talent. It also gives you another way to achieve the ultimate objective: to design a hairstyle that enhances your client's appearance. The key here is the minimal manipulation of the hair. If you blowdry the hair while moving it into place with your fingers, you will create a style that truly highlights the detailed texture within the razor cut.

These technical steps follow the client consultation, shampoo service, and haircut.

Procedure

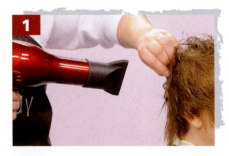

1 Apply a styling product of your choice and work it through the hair. Use your fingers and a blowdryer to gently move the textured hair into place. Use your fingertips to separate the textured ends. Notice the massaging action used to add texture and body while drying.

2 Use a small, rubber-based paddle brush to add fullness. In this style the lengths are turned up and forward toward the face.

© Milady, a part of Cengage Learning. Photography by Gary David Gold.

3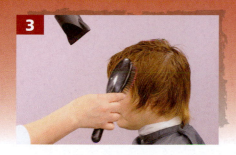

3 Use a paddle brush around the face to add length and direction. The brush will add polish to the lengths. Alternate the brush with the fingers to accentuate texture

4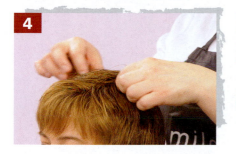

4 Use your fingertips to soften and personalize the design.

5 Finish with a combination of spray and blowdryer for added volume, separation, and texture.

6 The finished style is light and airy with soft fringe-like lengths around the face.

Create

Apply this technique to different hair lengths, colors, and textures for almost endless possibilities.

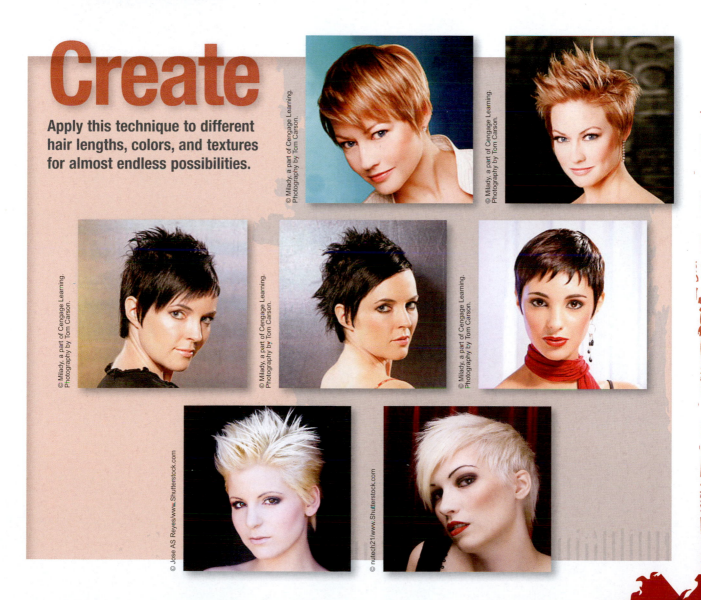

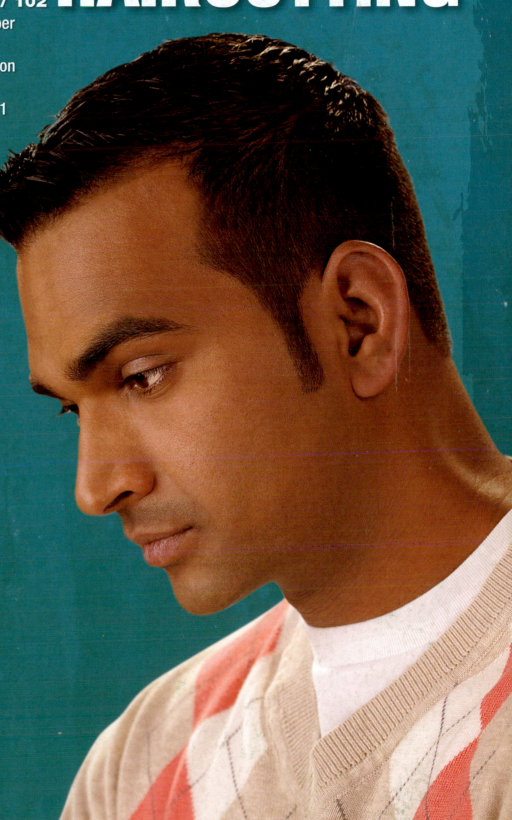

MEN'S HAIRCUTTING

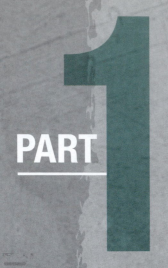

Layered Haircuts

The procedures you will use in men's layered haircutting are a fusion of barbering and cosmetology techniques that will serve you well in the salon. For example, you will learn how and why to hold your hands in certain positions as you work around the head, and you will learn about the elevations that allow you to retain or remove length while blending. Once mastered, these techniques will lead you to creating styles with a definitive male flair, instead of attempting to only use women's hair design principles on the male head form.

Another method frequently relied upon when performing layered cutting on men's hair is the use of the shear-over-comb technique to blend the sideburn, nape, and behind-the-ear areas. In this technique, you use the comb to position the hair to be cut while using the shears to remove length. This requires a steady hand and close attention to detail as these areas of the cut play a key role in the total look of men's hair design.

In general, men's haircutting techniques usually require shears with longer cutting blades. These shears allow you to remove more hair at a time and should have pointed rather than rounded tips to perform the fine tapering techniques and detail work required in men's haircutting. For men's haircutting, all-purpose and taper combs should be constructed with both close-spaced and wide-spaced teeth to provide versatility in combing, cutting tension, and the ability to blend from shorter to longer lengths of hair.

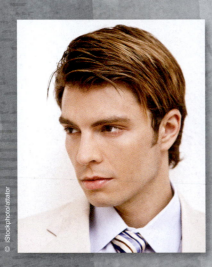

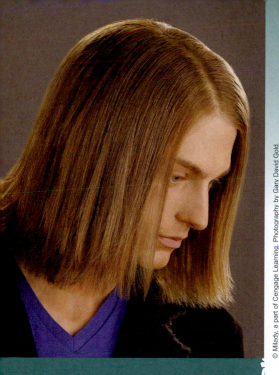

Long-Length Layers Haircut

Implements and Materials

You will need all of the following implements, materials, and supplies:

- **Cutting cape**
- **Neck strips**
- **Hair clips**
- **Spray bottle with water**
- **All-purpose comb**
- **Styling brush**
- **Shears**
- **Outliner**
- **Blowdryer**
- **Styling products**

Overview

With this first men's haircut, you will learn how to create designs by producing a more squared shape. As you remember from the women's haircutting part of this program, shapes for female cuts are generally more rounded and curved. Men's hairstyles are more often designed with a squared shape and form.

This long-layered silhouette provides textural movement and dimension. The combination of a perimeter guideline to establish the overall length and a traveling guide in the top section will be the reference points you use in creating long layers in the cut. These layers begin at nose level in the front and progress to longer lengths over the collar in the back section. Remember to mist the hair while cutting to maintain control.

These technical steps follow the client consultation and shampoo service.

This silhouette provides blended layers for a variety of long, texturized styles.

Technical Drawing

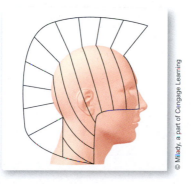

Long-Length Layers Haircut continued

Procedure

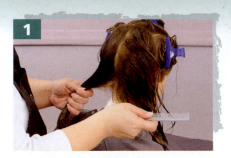

1 Begin this haircut by parting off the hair into five sections: a 2-inch (5cm) wide section from the front to crown in the top area and from ear-to-ear on the sides with two sections in the back.

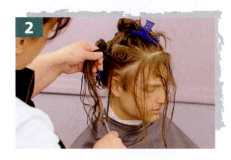

2 Part off a ½-inch (1.25 cm) subsection from around the hairline in each section, securing the remaining hair in each section with a clip.

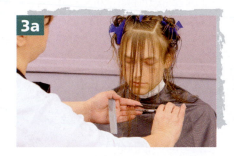
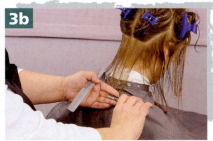

3 Comb the ½-inch (1.25 cm) parting down at 0-degree elevation, and create 1-inch (2.5 cm) wide guides at the center front and the center back.

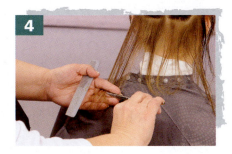

4 Start at the center back guide and use a horizontal finger position to cut the perimeter at 0 degrees until you have created a guideline that meets the front center guide.

Part 1: Layered Haircuts

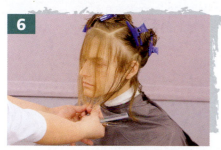

5 Repeat on the opposite side.

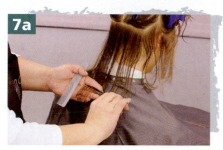

6 Check the sides for even length and the perimeter for blending. This perimeter guideline establishes the overall length of the cut.

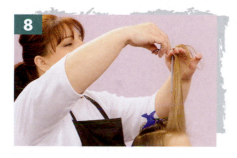

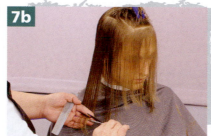

7 Starting at the left back section, bring down a ½-inch (1.25 cm) horizontal subsection. Cut to the perimeter guideline at 0-degree elevation. Then move to the right. Continue to take ½-inch (1.25 cm) subsections and cut to the guide until all hair on the sides and back is cut.

8 Release the top section and part off a ½-inch (1.25 cm) horizontal subsection from the front section. Hold the subsection at a 90-degree elevation and cut any stray hairs. Use this subsection as a traveling guide to cut the top section back to the center of the crown area.

9 Standing at the side, comb through and trim the top section at 90 degrees to blend the hair ends from the crown to front over the arc of the head.

Long-Length Layers Haircut continued

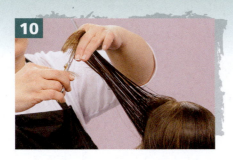

10 Take a ½-inch (1.25 cm) vertical subsection from the front of the left side and comb it at a 90-degree elevation. Use the perimeter guideline as a guide to cut and blend the subsection through the side up to the top section. The hair should blend with the top section in the recession or temple area. Check finger placement to make sure your fingers are straight and not curved when blending the panel and maintain even tension from the perimeter to the top section.

11 Repeat on the right side.

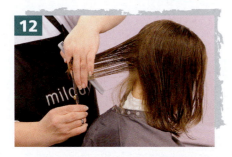

12 Continue taking vertical partings around the head form to blend from the perimeter through to the top section.

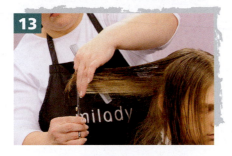

13 Standing behind the client, comb the hair back from the forehead and down on the sides and back. Comb through the side hair and include a section of the hair in back of the ears to make sure it blends with the back section.

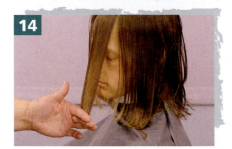

14 Check the perimeter to ensure a clean guideline, even length, and balance.

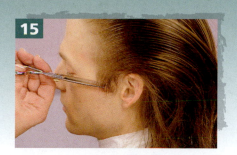

15 Comb the sides back out of the way to expose the sideburns. Cut the sideburns to the desired length and check the length in the mirror. If necessary, use the outliners to detail the bottom and back areas of the sideburn.

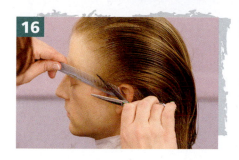

16 Starting at the bottom hairline of the sideburn, use the shear-over-comb technique to taper, blend, and remove excess fullness. Use the outliner to trim any unwanted neck hair in the nape area. For a finished look, apply the desired styling product, then finger-style or blowdry the hair.

Create

Apply this technique to different hair lengths, colors, and textures for almost endless possibilities.

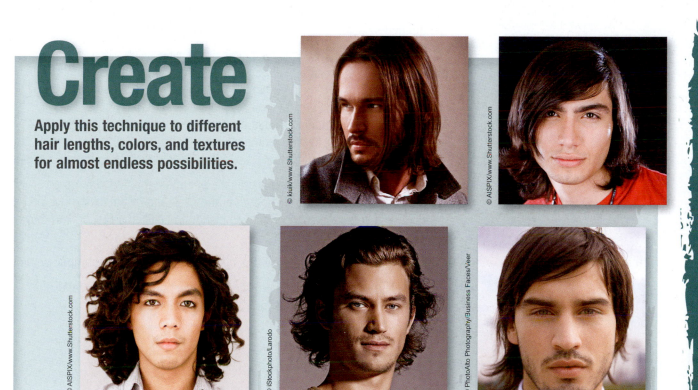

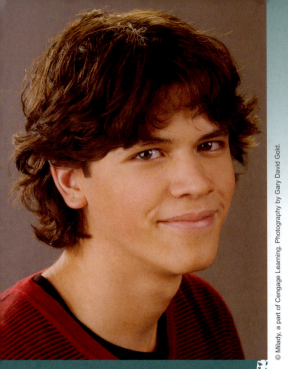

Medium- to Long-Length Layers Haircut

Implements and Materials

You will need all of the following implements, materials, and supplies:

- **Cutting cape**
- **Neck strips**
- **Hair clips**
- **Spray bottle with water**
- **All-purpose comb**
- **Styling Brush**
- **Shears**
- **Outliner**
- **Blowdryer**
- **Styling products**

Overview

This haircut begins with the long-length layer haircut you just created. You will now remove just enough length to create a medium-length layered shape. You will establish the perimeter guideline based on the client's desired length and by using facial features as reference points.

As in the previous haircut, hold the hair in a vertical position when cutting without overdirecting to maintain greater control of the lengths you are working with. For accuracy, part out ¼- to ½-inch (.6 to 1.25 cm) vertical sections when working with the perimeter as a guide to cut the internal layers of the top section. You will be creating a squared shape to accentuate and complement the male head shape. Avoid creating a curved or rounded shape as you cut by keeping your finger position straight and the client's head in an upright position.

The layered effect in this shape is created by cutting the perimeter to a medium- to long-length at the bottom of the neck and by establishing a long-length guide in the top section that will blend through the sides, up into the crest area.

These technical steps will follow the client consultation and shampoo service.

This medium-length silhouette provides long layers through the interior that extend almost to the perimeter for a young, casual look.

Technical Drawing

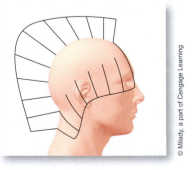

Procedure

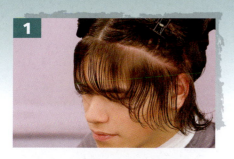

1 Part the hair into four sections, then part off a ½-inch (1.25 cm) subsection around the head.

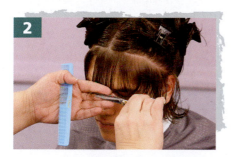

2 Establish the front length for the cut by using a reference point on the face.

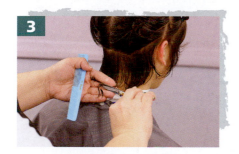

3 Establish a guide in the back using the neckline.

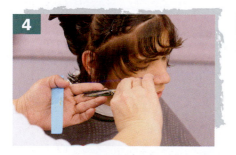

4 Use these guides to cut the perimeter guideline by connecting from one guide to the other.

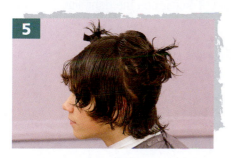

5 Release subsequent back and side partings and cut at 0-degree elevation to the perimeter guideline. Check the sides for even lengths.

Part 1: Layered Haircuts

Medium- to Long-Length Layers Haircut
continued

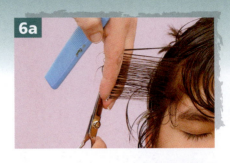

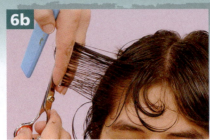

6 Part off a ½-inch (1.25 cm) vertical subsection from the right side and cut at a 90-degree elevation. Maintain vertical subsection while cutting through the side and crest.

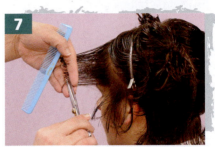

7 Repeat on the left side.

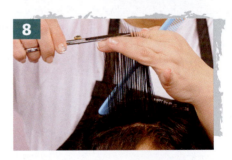

8 Use a horizontal traveling guide to cut the top section at a 90-degree elevation from the fringe to the crown, or from the crown to the front, making sure that the top section blends with the hair in the crest area. This will blend the top and side sections.

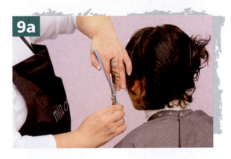

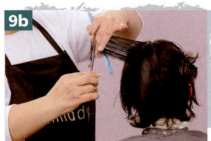

9 On the left side, use the hair previously cut directly behind the ear as a traveling guide. Cut vertical subsections at a 90-degree elevation, working toward the center back and up through the crown.

10 Repeat on the right side.

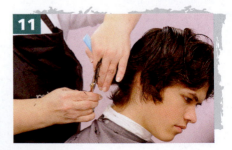

11 Check and fine-tune the blending from the sides through the back section by elevating hair sections at 90 degrees throughout the cut.

Part 1: Layered Haircuts

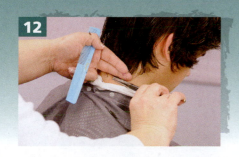

12 Check and fine-tune the guideline for evenness and a cleanly cut perimeter.

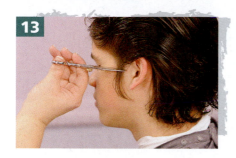

13 Comb the sides back out of the way to expose the sideburns. Using the mirror for accuracy, cut the sideburns to the desired length, blend with shear-over-comb technique, then detail using the outliners.

14 Use the outliner to trim any unwanted neck hair in the nape area.

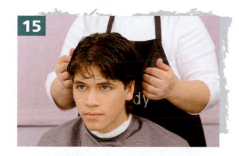

15 For finish, apply styling product and comb hair into desired style. Allow the hair to dry naturally or blowdry the hair into place starting in the back section and finishing in the top area.

Create

Apply this technique to different hair lengths, colors, and textures for almost endless possibilities.

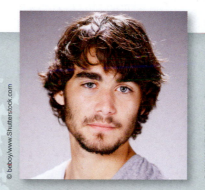

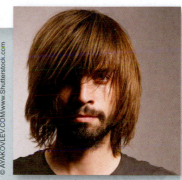

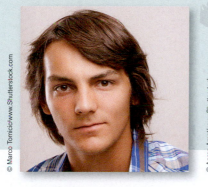

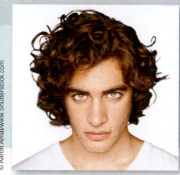

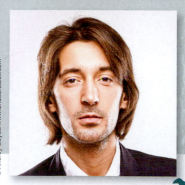

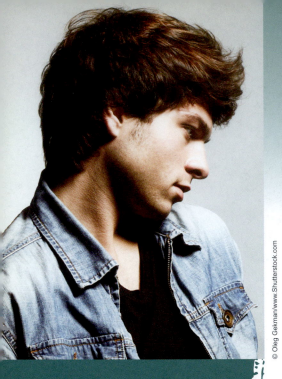

© Oleg Gekman/www.Shutterstock.com

Medium-Length Layers Haircut

Overview

Medium-length layered cuts tend to be uniformly cut in the top section and longer at the nape, with the back length just at or above the collar and with more fullness overall. This length of hair also requires that you pay attention to and work with the natural hairline in the nape area. Unlike the two previous haircut styles, this one is often blown dry to create the finished look. You will again be creating a squared shape to accentuate and complement the male head shape, so keep your finger position straight and the head in an upright position while cutting.

These steps follow the client consultation and shampoo service.

The layered effects in this shape provide texture and volume throughout the cut.

Technical Drawing

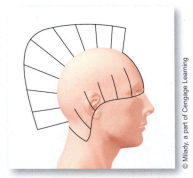

© Milady, a part of Cengage Learning

Procedure

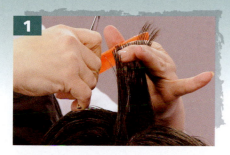

1 Begin this haircut by standing behind the client. This cut will use a five-section parting. Take a horizontal subsection 2- to 2½-inches (5 to 6.25 cm) wide at the top of the crown and cut to the desired length. Using this as your traveling guide, cut the entire top section, working your way towards the front hairline. Take a vertical subsection to check your cutting line.

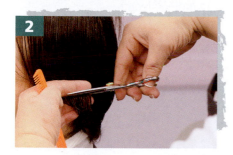

2 Move to the left side and comb the hair down to its natural falling position. Cut the side guideline to cover one-half to three-quarters of the ear, as the client desires. Repeat on other side.

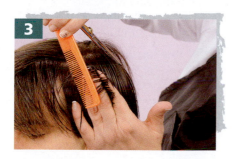

3 Standing behind the client, take a ½-inch (1.25 cm) vertical parting on the left side. Cut and blend the hair from the perimeter through the crest to the top section.

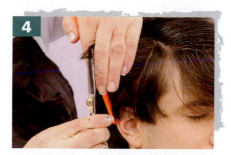

4 Repeat on the right side.

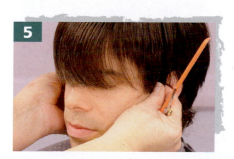

5 The top, crest, and sides should now be completely blended. Check sides for balance and evenness.

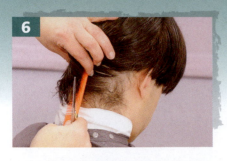

6 Part off a ½-inch (1.25 cm) subsection in the nape area and secure remaining hair with a clip as necessary.

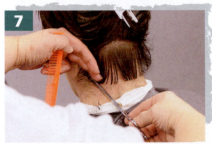

7 Starting in the center of the nape, create a guide length and then cut horizontally to the corners of the neck.

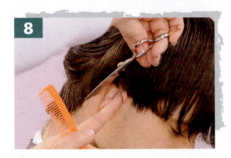

8 Move to the left side and cut the hair behind the ears to the nape corner to connect the sides and back sections on the perimeter guideline.

9 Repeat on the right side.

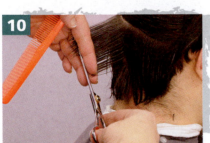

10 Take vertical partings from the nape guideline holding the hair at a 90-degree angle and cut up to the occipital bone. Move from the center of the nape through the left back section. Repeat right of center until the entire back section is cut.

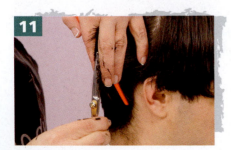

11 Take a ½-inch (1.25 cm) vertical parting from behind the ear, hold it straight out at 90 degrees, and cut to connect the perimeter guide to the top section. Repeat on the other side.

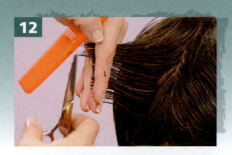

12 Check the haircut by combing horizontal sections held at a 90-degree angle from the sides into the back section to make sure the hair blends.

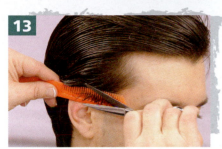

13 Comb the sides back out of the way to expose the sideburns. Cut the sideburns to the desired length, blend with the shear-over-comb technique, and then detail using the outliners.

14 Use the outliner to trim any unwanted neck hair in the nape area and to detail the guideline behind the ear.

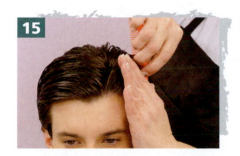

15 Apply styling product, comb hair into desired style, and allow to dry naturally; or, blowdry the hair, using a styling brush to turn the ends under in the nape and side areas before combing or brushing the sides back into the finished style.

Create

Apply this technique to different hair lengths, colors, and textures for almost endless possibilities.

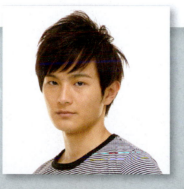

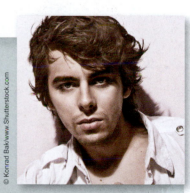

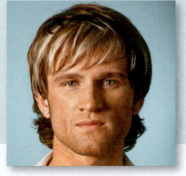

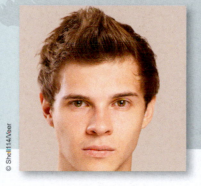

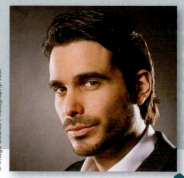

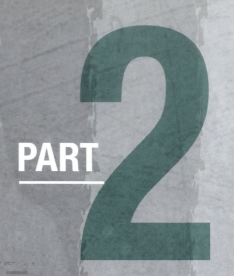

PART 2

Tapered Haircuts

Tapered haircut styles are shorter at the perimeter and get gradually longer through the crest and top sections. As you will see, the amount of tapering or how close to the scalp the hair is cut in the perimeter areas, along with how long the hair is left in the top and crest sections, is what differentiates one type of taper cut from another. These cuts will be performed using clippers, shears, razors, and/or outliners to accomplish a variety of different interior lengths, looks, and textures.

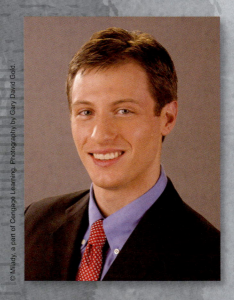

© Milady, a part of Cengage Learning. Photography by Gary David Gold.

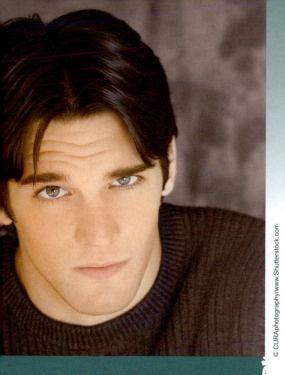

© CURAphotography/www.Shutterstock.com

Uniform Layers with Medium Taper Haircut

Implements and Materials

You will need all of the following implements, materials, and supplies:

- **Cutting cape**
- **Neck strips**
- **Hair clips**
- **Spray bottle with water**
- **All-purpose comb**
- **Styling Brush**
- **Shears**
- **Outliner**
- **Blowdryer**
- **Styling products**

Overview

This next haircut has uniformly layered top and side sections with a medium taper in the back section. The hair can be left long enough on the sides to cover part of the ear or cut shorter to expose the ears. Yet another variation is to cut the hair in uniform layers throughout to leave length at the perimeter in the nape area. This cut also creates texture and movement for versatile styling options such as swept-back styles, side parts, or naturally tousled looks as well.

These steps follow the client consultation and shampoo service.

This silhouette provides short layers that taper slightly at the nape to create a highly texturized and easy maintenance look.

Technical Drawing

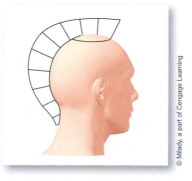

© Milady, a part of Cengage Learning

Uniform Layers with Medium Taper Haircut
continued

Procedure

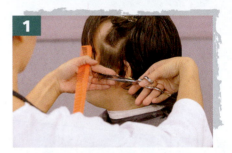

1 Begin this cut by determining how long to leave the hair on the sides using the hairline above the ears as a starting point. Take a ½-inch (1.25 cm) subsection and establish the perimeter guide length on both sides. Check both sides for balance and evenness.

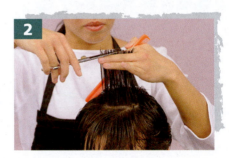

2 Stand behind the client and establish a 90-degree traveling guide length about 2–inches (5 cm) wide in the top section at the front of the crown. Cut the top section, working toward the face. Due to the shorter length of the hair, your hands will be closer to the head while cutting but avoid resting your hands against the head in order to control the angle of your fingers. Remember to not overdirect the hair partings while cutting in order to maintain the length of the hair.

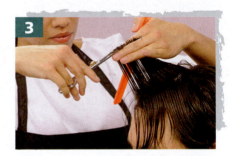

3 Standing at the side, check the top section you just cut by combing partings at 90 degrees from the crown over the arc of the head to the front and trim any ends that are not blended.

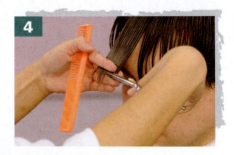

4 Comb the hair down in front and establish the front perimeter length.

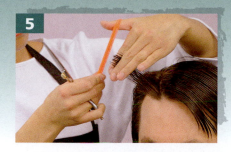

5 Again move in back of the client and comb the hair back from front to crown. Section off a vertical parting from the right front area of the crest that includes a portion of the top section, comb at a 90-degree elevation and cut to the top guide. On the right side of the head, you will be cutting to the top guide.

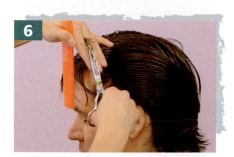

6 Repeat this step throughout the crest area until you reach the front section on the left side.

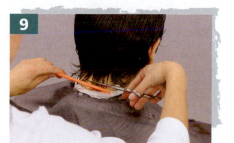

7 Move to the left side and comb down any subsequent partings and cut to the perimeter. Connect the side to the previously cut front guideline.

8 Repeat on the right side.

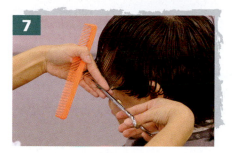

9 Move to the back section and establish the perimeter length, cutting subsequent parting lengths as necessary.

Uniform Layers with Medium Taper Haircut
continued

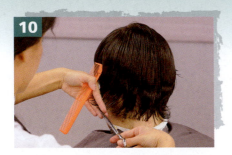

10 Beginning behind the left ear, cut the guideline behind the ear to the nape. Repeat on the right side.

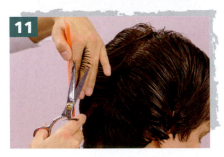

11 Next, section off vertical partings in the back at 90 degrees and use the perimeter guideline to cut and blend the hair from the perimeter to the crown area. Repeat until the entire back section has been cut.

12 Apply styling product if desired and finger-comb the hair for a texturized look. The use of a blowdryer and brush will create more volume that brings the hair strands together. As always, be guided by the client's desires and expectations for his final look.

Create

Apply this technique to different hair lengths, colors, and textures for almost endless possibilities.

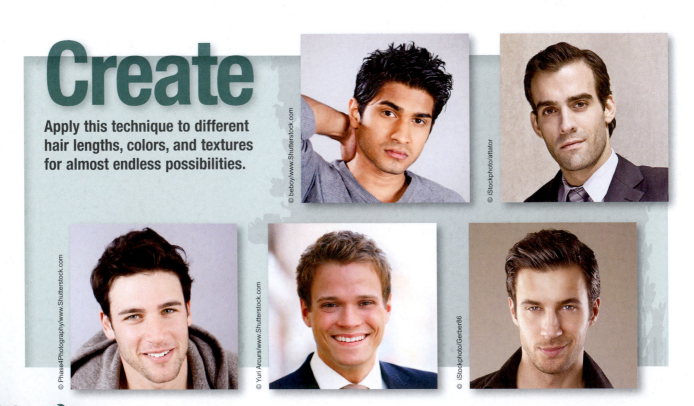

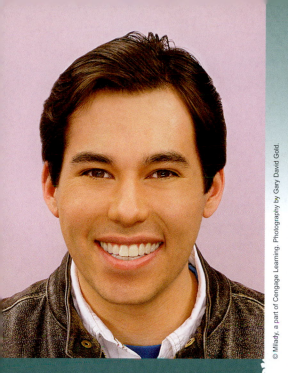

Combination Taper with Graduation Haircut

Implements and Materials

You will need all of the following implements, materials, and supplies:

- **Cutting cape**
- **Neck strip**
- **Hair clips**
- **Spray bottle with water**
- **All-purpose comb**
- **Styling Brush**
- **Shears**
- **Outliner**
- **Blowdryer**
- **Styling products**

Overview

This design emphasizes length and volume in the top, crest, and crown areas with most of the tapering being performed from the nape to the occipital area and around the ears at the hairline. The haircut will require the use of consistently elevated horizontal partings in the crest area and vertical partings, using diagonal finger placement, below the crest to create a balanced form. The result of these techniques will be seen in the weight that is created around the crest and into the side areas.

These steps follow the client consultation and shampoo service.

This silhouette is extremely popular with male clientele. Longer graduated interior lengths contrast with the shorter tapered perimeter that can be styled in a number of ways.

Technical Drawing

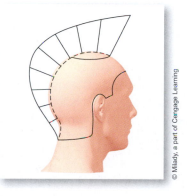

Combination Taper with Graduation Haircut
continued

Procedure

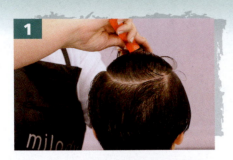

1 Part off the top section in a horseshoe shape that includes hair from the top of the crest through the crown.

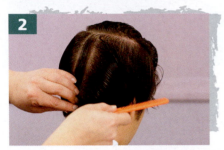

2 Begin by taking a vertical parting at the center of the back section, from the bottom of the crown to the nape.

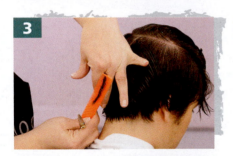

3 Starting at the nape, hold the section straight out from the head with a 45-degree finger placement from the nape to the occipital bone. Cut on the outside of your fingers to remove the hair that extends beyond your fingers.

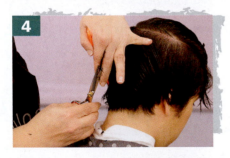

4 Move through the occipital area to the crown by gradually straightening your finger placement as you cut at a 90-degree elevation. As you reach the curve of the head through the occipital area this length will be your guide for the back and side sections. Continue taking vertical partings and cutting to the traveling guide as you work toward the front. Repeat on both sides.

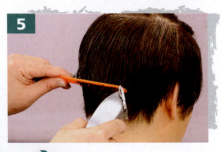

5 Move back to the nape and use your comb to position the hair for cutting with the clipper. Rest the comb against the head at about a 45-degree angle and use the clipper-over-comb technique to remove any excess length at the hairline. Check your previous shear work by using this technique to blend the hair from the nape to the occipital bone throughout the back section

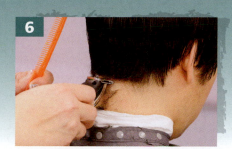

6 Use a free-hand technique with the outliner to finish the bottom of the hairline.

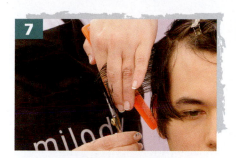

7 To graduate the shorter lengths around the ear use the perimeter line as a guide to position the fingers at a 45-degree angle from the hairline outward. Blend to the longer length in the crest area.

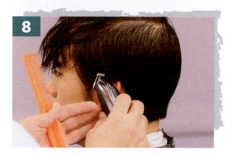

8 Combing the left side section back to expose the side hairline, position the outliner at about a 45-degree angle to trim around the ear. Repeat on the right side.

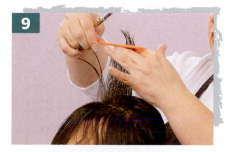

9 Release the top section of hair and comb it forward and down to section off a horizontal parting in the top section. Comb the parting at a 90-degree elevation, positioning the hair over your fingers to create a slight bevel, and establish a guide length.

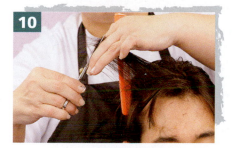

10 Finish the side section by blending the crest area to the top guide with the fingers placed at a 45-degree angle. Use the outliner to cut around and clean up the hair at the ear.

Combination Taper with Graduation Haircut
continued

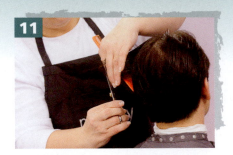

11 Repeat steps 9 and 10 on opposite side. When finished, the sides should look like a graduated 45-degree angle from the hairline to the crest.

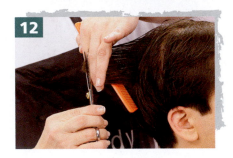

12 Work from front to back in a horseshoe pattern making sure the hair from the top and hair from the crest blends around the head and into the back section just below the crown.

13 The finished combination taper with graduation is symmetrical in nature. The longer weight area throughout the interior provides length and volume for styling versatility with a shorter perimeter hairline that is precisely contoured for a clean, refined look.

Create

Apply this technique to different hair lengths, colors, and textures for almost endless possibilities.

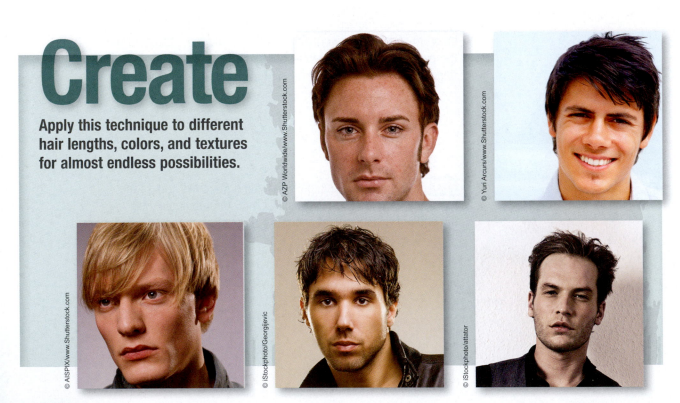

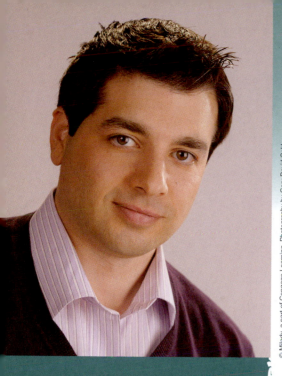

Contemporary Taper Haircut

Implements and Materials

You will need all of the following implements, materials, and supplies:

- **Cutting cape**
- **Neck strips**
- **Hair clips**
- **All-purpose and taper combs**
- **Styling Brush**
- **Shears**
- **Outliner**
- **Razor**
- **Styling products**

Overview

In this cut you will use your tapering techniques to fashion a medium-length look that sports volume, versatility, and a variety of finishing options. Paying close attention to detail work throughout this haircut results in a smooth finish that is sure to please. A moderately tapered neckline progresses to increasingly longer lengths through the interior for volume. This design is created using shears to remove length, an outliner to create detailed work, and razor work to create finely detailed transitions.

These technical steps will follow the client consultation and shampoo.

This cut is moderately close around the perimeter, progressing to longer lengths through the interior.

Technical Drawing

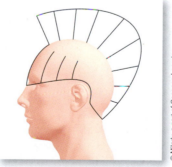

Contemporary Taper Haircut continued
Procedure

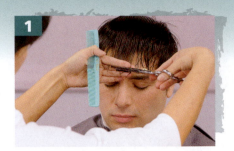

1 Comb the hair down in front and cut the front guide.

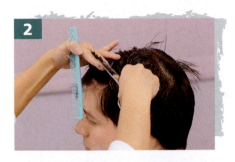

2 Comb the front guideline to position the hair at a 90-degree elevation. Comb through the parting again and slightly overdirect it toward the top of the head. Trim the ends to use this parting as the guide for the top section.

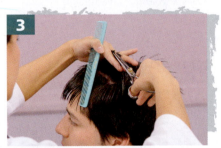

3 Cut top section starting at the front hairline and moving towards the crown.

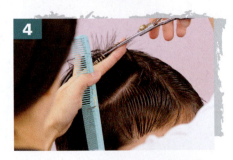

4 Cut and blend the crest area to the top guide around the entire head. Repeat on the opposite side of the top section.

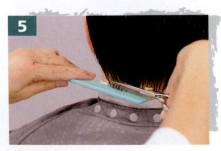

5 Next, section off a ½-inch (1.25 cm) parting at the hairline in the nape area. Begin at the center to establish the length at the nape and cut horizontally to the corners of the neck at 0-degree elevation to establish the guideline. Cut subsequent partings to this guideline.

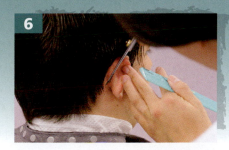

6 Next, move to the side and cut in the design line around the ear, then behind the ear so that the design line connects with the corner of the nape. Repeat on opposite side. Cut subsequent side partings from the bottom of crest down to the guideline on both sides.

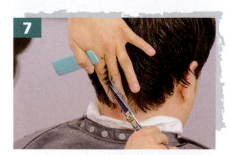

7 Using the guide at the nape, section off a ½-inch (1.25 cm) vertical parting from the center of the back holding it straight out from where it grows. Position your fingers at a 45-degree angle to gradually taper from the shorter lengths at the nape to the longer lengths at the crown. Note that your fingers will be gradually repositioned from the 45-degree angle to a straight vertical position as you cut through the entire back section to the crown.

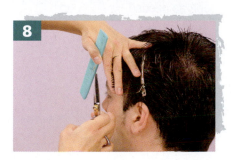

8 Use the same vertical parting and finger placement techniques used in the back section to blend the sides from the hairline to the top section. The length in the top section will determine the degree of the angle of your fingers that accommodates cutting from these shorter to longer lengths. As in the back section, be sure to maintain consistency in the tension, elevation, and finger placement of the hair when cutting the sides. Repeat on the opposite side of the head.

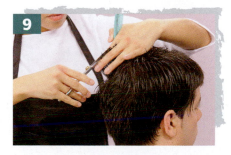

9 Comb through the entire cut, holding the hair at a 90-degree elevation, to check how well the cut blends from the top section to the hairline.

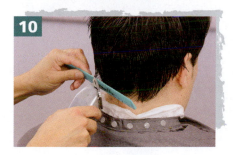

10 Use the clipper or shear-over-comb technique to remove any bulk and weight around or in back of the ear and in the nape area. Notice the angle at which the comb is held.

Contemporary Taper Haircut continued

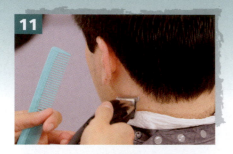

11 Refine the outer perimeter of the cut using the outliner with a comb or the free-hand technique.

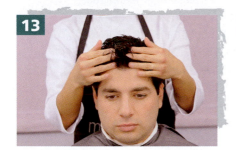

12 Check the haircut for even blending, then mist the hair in preparation for razor cutting. Use the razor rotation technique to blend the hair in crest and back transition areas. In this method, the comb and razor rotate to control and cut the hair. Note that you will need to hold the blade at slightly less than a 45-degree angle as it is run through the hair with a light touch to reduce any weight buildup. Work down toward the nape as needed.

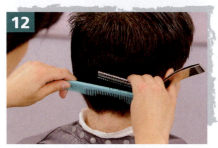

13 The length in the front provides a variety of styling options.

Create

Apply this technique to different hair lengths, colors, and textures for almost endless possibilities.

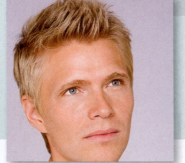

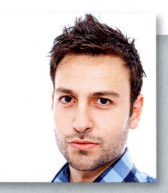

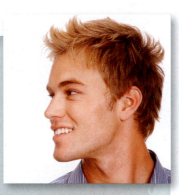

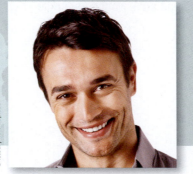

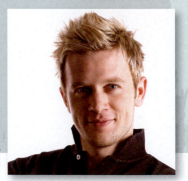

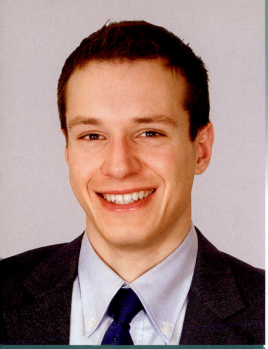

© iStockphoto/attator

Classic Taper Haircut

Implements and Materials

You will need all of the following implements, materials, and supplies:

- **Cutting cape**
- **Neck strips**
- **Hair clips**
- **Spray bottle with water**
- **All-purpose and taper combs**
- **Styling Brush**
- **Clippers**
- **Shears**
- **Outliner**
- **Blowdryer**
- **Styling products**

Overview

This classic tapered haircut will bring you to yet another level of expertise as you learn how to blend the transition areas within the interior sections. Being able to work with shears and clippers will help you create timeless looks that will always be in demand.

These technical steps follow the client consultation and shampoo.

This shape features a tapered perimeter that progresses into the uniformly layered rounded-off silhouette of the interior.

Technical Drawing

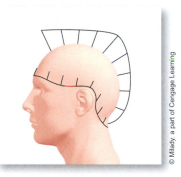

© Milady, a part of Cengage Learning

Classic Taper Haircut continued

Procedure

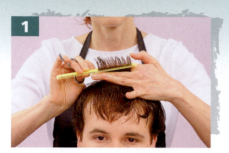

1 Take a horizontal parting at the front of the crown and cut the guide length for the top section, holding the hair at a 90-degree angle.

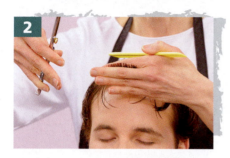

2 Working toward the front take thin, precise horizontal partings combed vertically at 90 degrees and cut the top section to the already established guideline length.

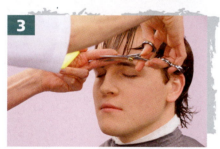

3 Comb the hair down in front and establish a front guideline.

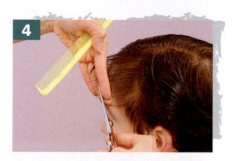

4 On the left side, pick up a vertical parting from the front recession area to use as a guide for the crest area. Cut the entire crest area from the front to crown, blending the hair to the top section. Repeat on the opposite side.

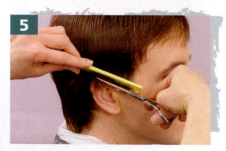

5 On the left side, create the guideline in front of the sideburns and around the ears. Repeat on the right side as shown.

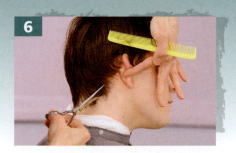

6 Cut subsequent partings from the side and behind the ear to the guideline and repeat on the opposite side.

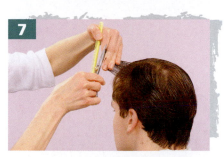

7 Use vertical partings at a 90-degree elevation to blend the hair on the sides from the guideline to the crest.

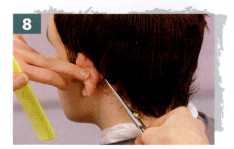

8 Move to center back section to establish the length and guideline at the nape. Cut horizontally to the left corner of the neck at 0-degrees elevation, then move to the side and connect the guideline from around the ear to the corner of the nape. Cut the guideline on the right side in the same way.

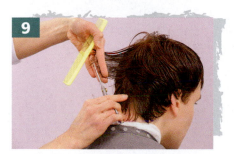

9 Using the guideline at the nape, take vertical partings held at a 90-degree angle and blend the hair from the hairline to the crown. Continue cutting vertical partings until the entire back section is cut.

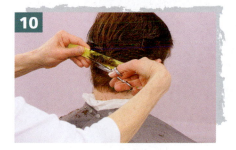

10 Follow-up the shear cutting in the back nape area with a shear-over-comb technique to taper below the occipital bone.

Classic Taper Haircut continued

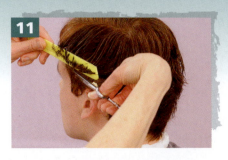

11 Continue this tapering technique around the perimeter over the ear area.

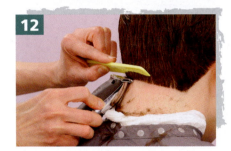

12 Use the clippers or outliners to create a clean perimeter line.

Create

Apply this technique to different hair lengths, colors, and textures for almost endless possibilities.

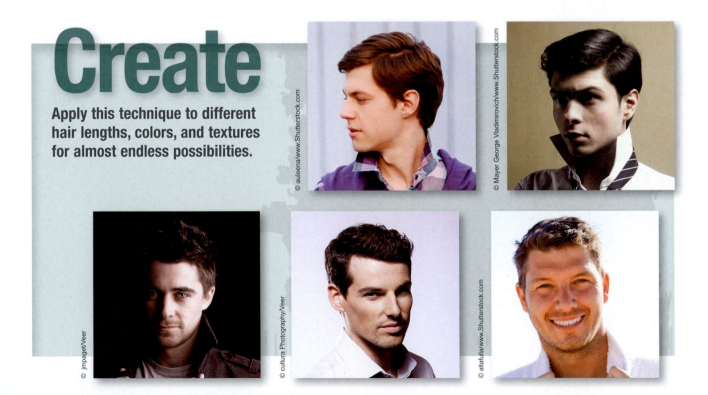

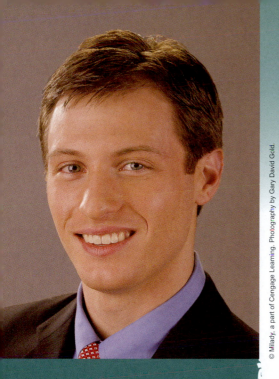

Gentlemen's Taper Haircut

© Milady, a part of Cengage Learning. Photography by Gary David Gold.

Implements and Materials

You will need all of the following implements, materials, and supplies:

- **Cutting cape**
- **Neck strips**
- **Hair clips**
- **All-purpose and taper combs**
- **Styling Brush**
- **Clippers**
- **Shears**
- **Outliner**
- **Styling products**

Overview

This shorter tapered look is ideal for the well-groomed businessman who prefers shorter lengths in the top section that convert easily from a recreational to a professional style for an always-groomed image. This style works well for several different face shapes and hair textures, including naturally curly or wavy hair. Note that no area is cut too short or extreme; instead, the look projects a well-balanced form as a result of the precision-cutting techniques used.

These technical steps follow the client consultation and shampoo.

This tapered cut features a slight elongation in the front of the top section to provide styling options.

Technical Drawing

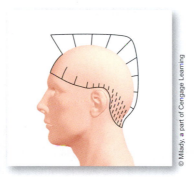

© Milady, a part of Cengage Learning

Gentlemen's Taper Haircut continued

Procedure

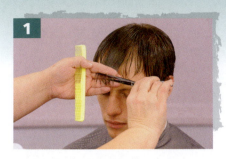

1 As with the previous haircut, comb the hair down in front and establish a guide length at 0-degrees elevation.

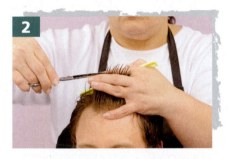

2 Standing in back of the client, comb the front guide to position the hair at a 90-degree elevation, again with slight overdirection to leave length. Trim the ends to use this parting as the guide for the top section.

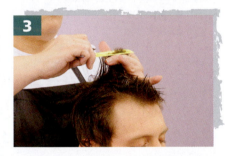

3 Cut the top section back to the crown.

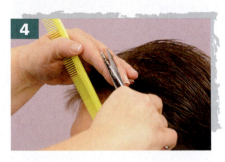

4 Return to the front section at the recession area for the next parting, combing it straight up from where it grows. Cut to the top guide. Continue to cut subsequent partings through the crest to the center of the crown.

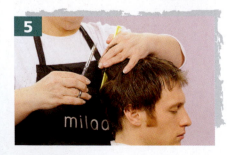

5 Repeat on the opposite side of the head, working to the crown. Note that the hair lengths should meet in the center of the crown.

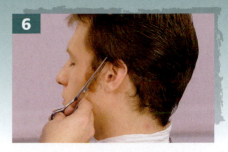

6 Next, section off a ¼-inch to ½-inch (.6 to 1.25 cm) parting at the hairline in front of the sideburns and around the ear. Cut the guideline.

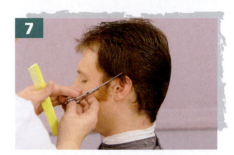

7 Cut subsequent partings to the guideline and repeat on the opposite side.

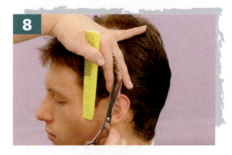

8 Use vertical partings, held at a 90-degree angle, to blend the hair on the sides from the guideline to the crest.

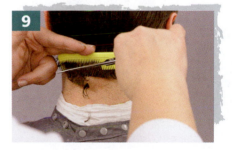

9 Move to center back section and establish the length and guideline at the nape. Cut horizontally to the corners of the neck at 0-degrees elevation, then move to the side and connect the guideline from around the ear to the corner of the nape. Cut subsequent partings to the guideline and repeat on the opposite side.

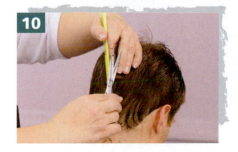

10 Using the guideline at the nape as a reference, take vertical partings held at 90 degrees and blend from the hairline to the crown. Continue cutting vertical partings until the entire back section is cut.

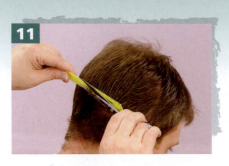

11 Use the shear-over-comb technique to further taper the sides and back, being careful not to cut too deeply.

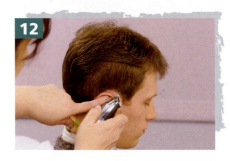

12 Refine and detail the cut using an outliner, then style the hair into place for a perfect business look.

© Milady, a part of Cengage Learning. Photography by Gary David Gold.

Create

Apply this technique to different hair lengths, colors, and textures for almost endless possibilities.

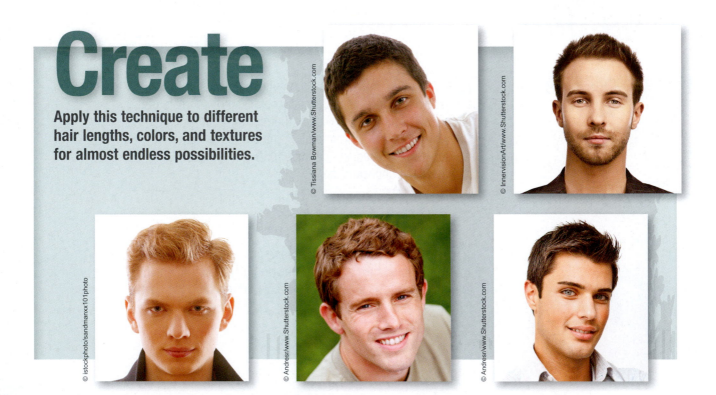

© Tissiana Bowman/www.Shutterstock.com

© InnervisionArt/www.Shutterstock.com

© istockphoto/sandmanxx101photo

© Andresr/www.Shutterstock.com

© Andresr/www.Shutterstock.com

PART

3 High Taper Haircuts

High taper cuts are very short through the nape and sides with short, layered lengths in the top section. Haircut styles such as the *Flat-Top, Crew Cut, Brush Cut*, and *Fades* are all variations of high taper cuts. Very short graduation creates a "faded" look at the perimeter with gradually increasing length through the crest and into the top section. The overall finish of these types of cuts shows smooth transitions from one section of the head form to another. Accuracy and skill are needed to create these cuts so that the design complements the client's head shape and facial features. With experience, your eye will tell you if a cut is proportionate for the client.

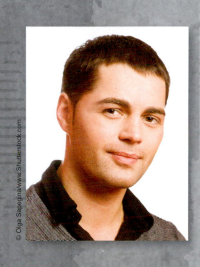

© Olga Sapegina/www.Shutterstock.com

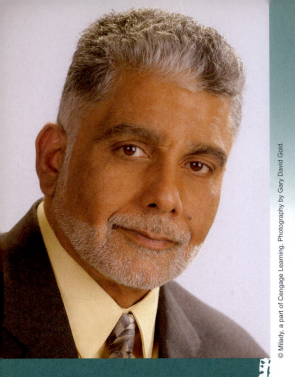

Short Brush Haircut

Implements and Materials

You will need all of the following implements, materials, and supplies:

- **Cutting cape**
- **Neck strips**
- **Hair clips**
- **Spray bottle with water**
- **All-purpose and taper combs**
- **Styling Brush**
- **Clippers**
- **Shears**
- **Outliner**
- **Blowdryer**
- **Styling products**

Overview

This men's haircut produces shorter lengths at the nape progressing to longer lengths at the top of the head. This is a versatile and popular design that offers styling options and easy maintenance.

This haircut requires free-hand clipper, clipper-over-comb, and shear cutting. You will also want to fine-tune your shear-over-comb coordination to master the blending techniques needed for this cut.

These technical steps follow the client consultation and shampoo.

This short, dynamic shape features a closely tapered perimeter with short lengths through the back and sides that gradually blend to a top length between 1 and 1½ inches (2.5 to 3.75 cm).

Technical Drawing

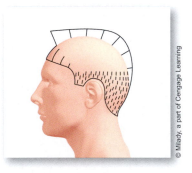

Procedure

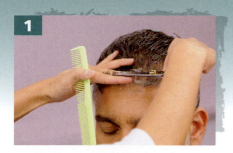

1 Beginning at the front hairline, comb the hair straight up at a 90-degree elevation and establish a traveling guide.

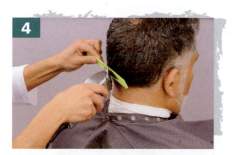

2 Cut from the front through the top section to the crown area.

3 Move to the back section and use the free-hand clipper technique with the blades open to cut the first inch (2.5 cm) of hair from the hairline to the back section.

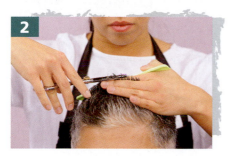

4 Switch to the clipper-over-comb technique to cut from the lower nape section up to bottom of the crest. Cut the left side first, then repeat on the right side.

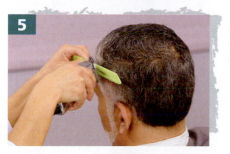

5 Continue to use free-hand clipper and clipper-over-comb techniques to cut the sides. Start on the left. Cut only to the bottom of the crest, which should be in line with the temple. Repeat on the right side.

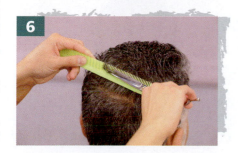

6 Next, use shear-over-comb cutting to blend the hair at the crest with the top section around the entire head. Note that it is very important to hold the still blade parallel to the base of the comb when cutting. The thumb moves the cutting blade.

Short Brush Haircut continued

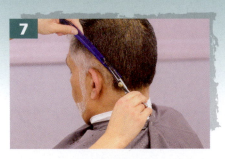

7 Use a barbering or tapered comb to create the final details of the finished taper at the nape and around the ears. The taper comb allows you to cut the hair shorter and closer at the lower part of the perimeter hairline and makes cutting the nape, the sideburns, and the ear area easier.

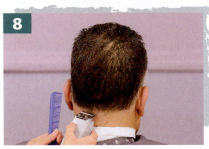

8 To detail the sideburns, around the ears, and behind the ears use a free-hand technique with the outliner. Use the outliner to create a sharp perimeter line at the nape.

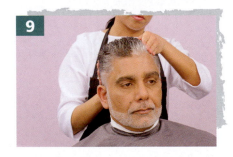

9 The finished brush cut can be styled using products or combed into place and allowed to dry naturally.

Create

Apply this technique to different hair lengths, colors, and textures for almost endless possibilities.

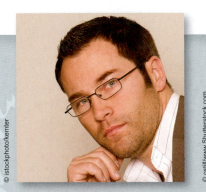

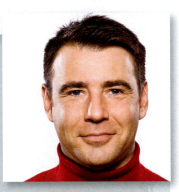

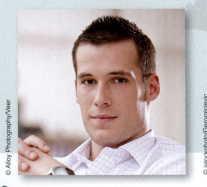

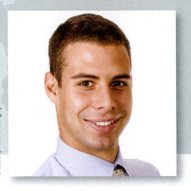

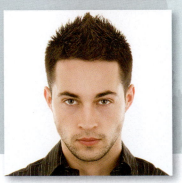

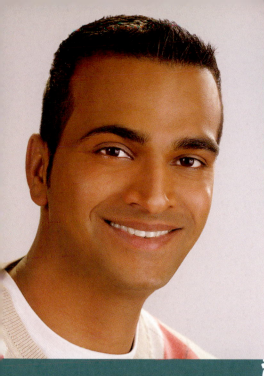

Close Taper Haircut

Implements and Materials

You will need all of the following implements, materials, and supplies:

- **Cutting cape**
- **Neck strips**
- **All-purpose and taper combs**
- **Natural bristle brush**
- **Clippers**
- **Outliner**
- **Styling products**

Overview

There are many variations of short taper styles; however, all require attention to detail and precise blending with the clippers. Like other haircut styles, the crest is a transition area from the top to the sides, and it is in this section of the head form where the length of the hair tends to vary the most. This is because close cutting in the crest area can begin at the bottom, mid-point, or at the top of the crest. The key is to clearly understand what the client wants in his finished look.

These technical steps follow the client consultation and shampoo.

This short, dynamic shape features a closely tapered perimeter with very short lengths through the back and sides that gradually blend to a very short length in the top section.

Technical Drawing

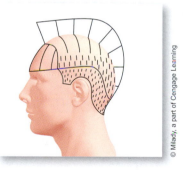

Close Taper Haircut continued

Procedure

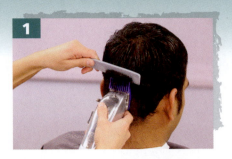

1 Begin at the center of the nape section. Using clippers with a #4 guard, cut the center back section in a vertical panel to the bottom of the crest.

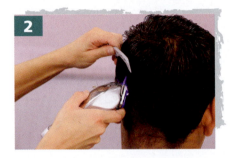

2 Cut in the sections left and then right of center in the same manner.

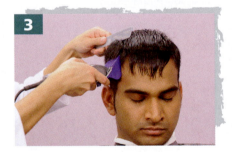

3 Move to the right side and use a #2 guard to cut from the hairline to the bottom, middle, or top of the crest as the client desires. This will create a "line" of hair around the crest area.

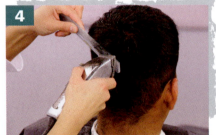

4 Next, remove the guard and open the clipper blades a notch. Beginning at the bottom of the line you created at the ear, use the clipper-over-comb technique to blend the weight line around the head.

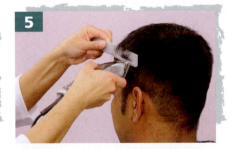

5 Next, open the blades completely and blend the hair from the crown to the top section, then at a slight diagonal through the crest areas. Repeat on the opposite side.

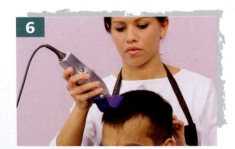

6 Attach a #9 guard and blend the hair through the top section.

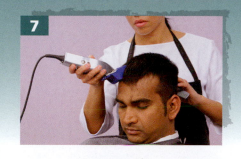

7 Continue working down through the crest by closing the blades slightly as you blend the hair into the crest areas.

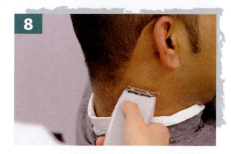

8 Once the cut is completely blended and faded, use the outliner to perform detailing work around the hairline.

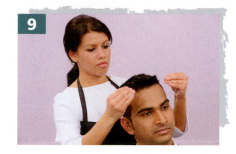

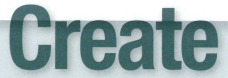

9 Finish with a styling aid as the client desires.

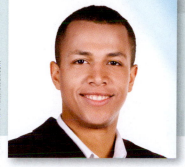

Create

Apply this technique to different hair lengths, colors, and textures for almost endless possibilities.

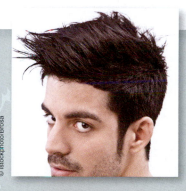

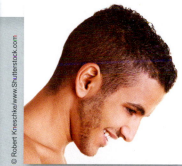

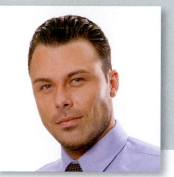

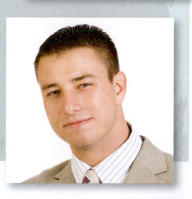

Notes

Notes

Notes

Notes

Notes

Notes

Notes

Notes

Notes

Notes

Notes